Sweet Sixteen
with Hodgkin's

I started reading *Sweet Sixteen*... and couldn't put it down! If you haven't had the luxury of meeting or interacting with Molly Jodeit at some time in your life, then being able to read and learn from her life experiences is an invaluable opportunity. One of the hardest things in medicine is the delivery of bad news to a patient; especially to a young, happy, and an otherwise unencumbered individual when you know that this will change their life forever!

The positive way in which Molly and the entire Jodeit family accepted this challenge combined with their strong religious faith has touched many who know them. The story of this brave young woman's cancer journey is outlined in the book. Observing Molly's courage and positive attitude in dealing with adversity has certainly touched my life and left me changed.

> —James E. Muntz, M.D. Clinical Professor of Medicine, Clinical Associate Professor of Orthopedics, Baylor College of Medicine; team physician for Houston Texans, Rockets, and Houston Astros

The theme in this book is God's sovereignty... and the way His glory shines forth each day. This book is a glimpse of how God works in our lives everyday and how important our Faith in Him is. Molly's illness was the reason this book was initiated, and throughout it you will see what a sweetheart she is. Everyday, I looked forward to reading about God and the mighty work he was doing in Molly's life. I am thankful that this illness was cured... she fought a gallant battle and I love her and am proud of her.

> —Ed A. Smith, former Chairman of the Board of the YMCA; Chairman Emeritis, Center for Hearing and Speech, and most important of all, Molly's grandfather

This is a book of hope! When the frightening storm of cancer blew through the lives of the Jodeit Family, they ran to God for shelter. You will see His hand at every turn and will be encouraged as you read the simply stated devotionals and conversations of dear friends who walked beside them and prayed for them. It is a testament to God's grace and His Glory. Cathy's openess will help you through the times when nothing is left except a stark faith in God.

—Roger Wernette, Executive Director of The Gathering of Men in Houston and Cathy's Sunday school teacher, CEPC

I was inspired by the steadfast faith so clearly expressed in person by this family during those difficult months of Molly's cancer treatment and now in Cathy Jodeit's heartfelt book *Sweet Sixteen with Hodgkin's* about their family's journey. It is clear to me that Molly was helped tremendously by the foundation, rock if you will, of confidence and spiritual strength that Mel and Cathy provided throughout her treatment. This book is a reflection of the faith in God they embrace and the hope in God that they stand on. This story is about Molly, a remarkable young adult who faced uncertainty and a scary disease with unflinching courage week after week. As with all young people who are forced to walk this path, life takes on new meanings and undoubtedly this journey will make her an even better person. It is a privilege to be her doctor and I too am thankful for the guidance I receive from God.

—Kenneth McClain M.D. Ph.D, Texas Children's Hospital.

Sweet Sixteen
with Hodgkin's

*A mom's story of holding God's hand
through trials & triumphs*

written by:
Catherine Jodeit

TATE PUBLISHING *& Enterprises*

Sweet Sixteen with Hodgkin's
Copyright © 2007 by Cathy Jodeit. All rights reserved.

This title is also available as a Tate Out Loud product. Visit www.tatepublishing.com for more information.

No part of this publication may be reproduced, stored in a retrieval system or transmitted in any way by any means, electronic, mechanical, photocopy, recording or otherwise without the prior permission of the author except as provided by USA copyright law.

Scripture quotations marked "NIV" are taken from the *Holy Bible, New International Version* ®, Copyright © 1973, 1978, 1984 by International Bible Society. Used by permission of Zondervan Publishing House. All rights reserved.

The opinions expressed by the author are not necessarily those of Tate Publishing, LLC.

Published by Tate Publishing & Enterprises, LLC
127 E. Trade Center Terrace | Mustang, Oklahoma 73064 USA
1.888.361.9473 | www.tatepublishing.com

Tate Publishing is committed to excellence in the publishing industry. The company reflects the philosophy established by the founders, based on Psalms 68:11,
"The Lord gave the word and great was the company of those who published it."

Book design copyright © 2007 by Tate Publishing, LLC. All rights reserved.
Cover design by Liz Mason
Interior design by Sarah Leis

Published in the United States of America

ISBN: 978–1–6024734–4-7
1. Christian Inspiration   2. Surviving Cancer

07.07.24

This journal has been compiled to honor the Mighty God whom we serve. He has shown His Glory, been faithful to His word, and been victorious through this battle. His grace will forever enfold us, His mercies fall down upon us and His Love will ever uphold us. We give thanks to His glorious name.

Acknowledgemnts

It is with my heartfelt love and appreciation that I extend my gratitude to my dear friend Kitty Kyle. She took the initiative from the very beginning of Molly's journey and prayerfully shared our story. She forwarded the emails I had sent her of my heart's conversations with God, my specific prayers of praise and concerns and my fears and joys. She was a constant, stable source of encouragement through uplifting words, selected devotionals and forwarded replies of friends to the e-mails which were sent. She enabled an invaluable communication of support for Molly and all of us as we helped Molly to tackle this day to day challenge.

Thank you, Kitty, for jumping on the train, without hesitation, and going down the tracks with us.

May our Mighty God Bless you always for the initiative you took to encourage us through this journey. As a cancer survivor yourself, you knew of the encouragement we would need. We are forever grateful!

In Christ's Love,
Cathy

Contents

13	Foreword
15	Introduction
17	The Beginning
31	Phase I: The Battle Begins
69	The Fight Continues
96	The Final Round
145	Phase II: On to Radiation
209	It is Finished
230	Afterword

Foreword

Just a little bit about our family...

We are a close Christian family, all living in Houston and we see each other quite often. Mel and I have been blessed with four precious children, three daughters and one son. Our two oldest daughters are married and we have one grandson and another one on the way. Molly is our youngest.

These reflections, prayers and lessons are heartfelt concerns about our Molly. She was 16 years old and a sophomore in high school, when she was diagnosed with Cancer, Hodgkin's Lymphoma, Stage 4. Though she is the one with cancer, for those of you who have experienced this world of cancer, you know it truly affects the whole family.

Life is fragile and we count our blessings and thank God for His strength, His wisdom, and His protection as we weathered this storm. We especially thank Him for what He did to and through Molly. She is a beautiful, gentle spirited and sweet natured warrior; she has a love for life, an eye for style and balance, and a unique ability to categorize good from bad, yesterday from today, what needs to be done and doesn't and move on!

Molly was born seven years after our other three children and though she has been influenced by all of us, she has managed to be an independent young adult with defined ambitions. She is very private and her consent to let me share her story is truly her gift to me and hopefully to the many who will read it.

Praise God wherever you are and whatever situation He has allowed you to be in, for His Glory will shine through.*

PRAISE!

*This is a thought that was put on my heart at the beginning of this journey. It remains the signature of each e-mail sent from my computer. I have learned to appreciate the significance of EACH word included in its content but especially the first one.

Introduction

These e-mails and various replies (there were too many to include all of them) that I have compiled will take you through our journey of Molly's cancer from beginning to end. I did feel like I was holding God's hand...I was desperate for His presence, His continued reminder that He was in charge, and I needed His strength. This was my youngest, one of my precious daughters and as a mom I wanted it to be me not her...She was too young...I could handle it better...And she is sixteen, such a formidable age...I wanted to protect her and I couldn't!

I found out through this journey that this child is strong...she is capable and she had the ability to do what needed to be done and not ponder on it when it was over. I have learned invaluable lessons by watching her as she daily tackled this disease. Yes, she was the gentle warrior but this gentle warrior fought a courageous battle. She was flanked by the prayers of other warriors all over the country and it was amazing to watch as one by one the dragon challenges were slain.

When you read these, please, don't look at details, look at the content. Someone said, "I felt like I was having a cup of coffee with you at the kitchen table when I would read your e-mails." I am pretty "down home!" No fancy words, or perfect grammar, a bunch of dot dot dots, and exclamations marks and simple stories that many of you will relate to.

Just sit with me a while and have a cup of coffee and enjoy these e-mails...my hope is that God will use them to encourage some of you who are facing tough trials... the lessons God gave me were not isolated to CANCER; they are lessons that can be used for any of us, for any challenge... no matter how big or small. May you find comfort, encouragement, and hope as you read them. We serve a mighty God who has offered to be by our side... But He will not intrude... He is a gentle spirit who knocks softly and waits to be invited in.

Thank you for picking this book up. I know how many "reads" are out there and I pray that God will touch your heart in his loving way as your read our story... or God's story, and that you will be able to incorporate some of these lessons into your own lives.

Praise God wherever you are and whatever situation He has allowed you to be in, for His Glory will shine through.

The Beginning

Monday, March 13th was when it all started... actually this disease had been working hard behind the scenes for months... but that Monday was when it was brought to light.

Molly is 16, a sophomore in high school. She is our youngest daughter, the third daughter of four children. In July 2006, Molly had a small swollen lymph gland and I took her to see our GP named Dr. James Muntz. It was a minor infection and was treated with antibiotics. So a few months later when she felt like her neck was swollen, I obviously didn't take it as seriously as I should have! It didn't hurt and was more of a swollen place that a lump. She had been playing a lot of tennis and I just let it go. We were on Spring Break weeks later and Molly was rubbing her neck, "Dad, there is this thing on my neck and really bothers me..." He was on the phone on Friday am when we got back to town. The earliest appointment was Monday morning at 8:30. Molly and I were there. We were sent for a contrast cat scan at 10:30 and by 1:30 Dr. Muntz was on the phone with the following words:

"We have gotten back the results and Cathy, she has lymphoma." I had heard the term but had no idea what it meant.

"What is that", I asked?

"It is cancer."

"Cancer? She is sixteen! We don't have any of that in our family! How could she have cancer?" (Then I know there must have been a long pause...) and I asked, "Where do we even begin?"

"We have got to decide which cancer facility would be the best fit for her and who will be the best Doctor to treat her", Muntz said, and then he added: "Do you want to call Mel (my husband) or do you want me too?"

"You please, he will ask questions that I wouldn't think of."

Meantime, after Mel talked to Dr. Muntz, we all huddled by the phone for the next two hours to find the right doctor and the right hospital. Dr. Muntz was working from his contacts, I was working from mine... starting with my dad who made several calls gathering information from his trusted doctors. This was his grand daughter... He was devastated as well! He just kept saying, "I can't believe this!" I couldn't either... None of us could.

Both avenues led straight to Dr. David Poplack, M.D., Chief of Texas Children's Hematology-Oncology Service at Texas Children's Hospital in Houston. Calls were made and we had an appointment with Dr. Kenneth McClain, M.D., Ph.D. a well respected doctor in Dr. Poplack's group known for his research and excellence in the oncology field especially focusing on research for a disease called Histiocytosis. He would turn out to be our greatest adversary and friend. God had gone before us!

I remember picking Molly up at school on that Monday afternoon, watching her laughing and talking with friends and thinking: her life will forever be changed after today!

I told her the diagnosis on the way home and her one question was, "Am I going to die?"

"NO, you are not, God is going to fight this with us... and we are going to get it!" She was quiet the rest of the way home. I can't imagine the fury of emotions that she kept so closely guarded within her heart.

"We have got to see what we are dealing with" said McClain, and surgery was scheduled for Wednesday. This would not be a needle biopsy because they needed more tissue to run accurate tests. She would have part of this tissue removed from her neck as well as bone marrow from both of her hips. She went in at 11:00 am and we were home the same day at 9:30 pm. This was Wednesday. The Thursday following, she had to be at the Great Houston Imaging Center (GHIC) at 8:00 a.m. for additional tests. She would get a PET test and another CT scan. These tests would determine the location of this disease.

Let me just make a note here: We (Mel and I) gave this to God as soon as we heard. (Like God didn't already have it!) This is devastating news. We asked dear friends and family to be praying for Molly. Protect her from fear and give wisdom to those who have been chosen to take care of her.

On Wednesday I had to call GHIC and confirm the tests to be given on Thursday. I talked directly to Cynthia, the diagnostician, and asked what preparation they would need to do to Molly before the tests, explaining that she is so afraid of needles. Cynthia said since Molly is so scared of shots and pricks, ask TCH to leave in the line that they used for surgery. They will not want to do it, but fight for it, for we have a 50/50 chance that that line might work for tomorrows tests and it would save her the trauma of being stuck again. Whoever heard of such a thing! We prayed and we asked and they did it; the line worked the next day! God was doing that at every turn.

How were we able to have a surgery scheduled so quickly? They did it!

On Friday, March 17th, Molly was specifically diagnosed with Hodgkin's Lymphoma, Phase 4 A.

My other children were shaken completely. Jamie Ann "happened" to be at the hospital on the same day that we went to see Dr. Muntz for Molly's initial appointment. She was taking her 2 month old baby for a check–up. When we finished the CT scan, I called Jamie and asked her if she was still in the building and she said yes. She came over with the baby and met up with Molly and me. There was still no indication that this was serious except by a strange expression that I noticed on Dr. Muntz's face when he examined her neck and... he seemed quieter than usual. He tried to lighten it up by asking Molly what she had planned for the summer. When she said she wanted to do something fashion related, he told her he knew of a wonderful lady and friend of his who owned a cosmetic company and he could make a call and maybe he could help her get an internship. That got her wheels thinking about something other than what we were really here for. What a wise and thoughtful doctor and friend. He told her to send him a resume and he would forward it on.

I had to go to a short meeting that same day at 11:00 for the Center for Speech and Hearing. It was a follow up meeting to tie up some loose ends after an event that Mel and I had just chaired honoring my Dad and his brother Weldon. So Jamie and Molly and the baby went on to lunch at Barnaby's and talked about fashion and what to put on her resume and what she wanted to really do with fashion etc. They had a fun lunch and then Jamie took her back to school.

I had gotten back home about noon and had a little time to be still and quiet, reflect on the morning and what was to come… that is when I went to the garage and sat on the igloo! (A story later will relate to that.) Jamie came by the house a little later to check to see if there was any news… and she stayed for a while. The phone rang around 1:30 and this part is sort of a blur. This is what Jamie says happened: I was standing at the window looking out at the backyard, talking and she heard the word cancer, but she didn't think that is was about Molly because I was too calm. She was already tearing up because she was scared. She said she continued to watch and she listened and heard, "where do we go from here?" I got off the phone and said, "Molly has cancer!"

She said she couldn't believe it and was so puzzled by my calmness. You see, God was there… He knew what the day was to hold and he also knew I would need Him to hold me but especially that I would ask Him to hold our precious Molly close and in his arms! The tears came but they came gently… She is only 16… I thought… she is just too young for such a battle.

Jennifer, my oldest daughter was at work when we called her. It hit her hard as well for this was the littlest sister, the one they messed with and teased, not one who would have to take on something "Big" like cancer! She went straight to the computer and dove in looking for any possible information on Hodgkin's and treatments etc. She tried to stay at work but emotionally was totally distracted and ended up having to leave early. With info in hand, she left and began a mission to gather a bunch of camouflage things, a darling huge "camo" purse, some books, a cool pen, etc. and brought them home to Molly and said, "The theme is fight, fight, fight".

There were a few tears from everyone...but Molly was the strong one. Jon, Jennifer's husband joined us that night after work and Jamie Ann and her husband, Blake came by as well...This news just shook all of our lives up. You could already see the forces joining though. We are a strong family, and when a battle arose, we knew how to unite. The battle was here!

Tom, our son, was living with us while working and going to law school. He was in Destin, Florida on Spring Break when we called and told him about Molly. It must have hit him pretty hard too because a friend who was on this trip recognized that something was really wrong with him and pulled him aside and said "what's going on?" After he told her, they talked it through and prayed about it. Tom was still reeling from the news. Then a friend, who "happened" to be on Spring Break with him and was staying in the same house, was pulled into the conversation because she had battled cancer at young age herself and was a survivor. It had been several years ago and she had fully recovered. That gave Tom something definitive that he could hang his thoughts on. If she had fought her lymphoma successfully then Molly too could tackle this...but he had to talk to her. So he called Molly and asked her how she was and told her of the friend he had just talked to and how she had conquered her cancer several years ago. The conversation was appreciated and I think it gave Molly a measure of comfort...someone else around her age had walked down this road...and it worked!

Just as life is, everybody was in their spot...but this news hit all of our neat little structured worlds. Each of us would have our own roles...but each of us would have a role...We would rally; what ever it took...we would rally!

The following Monday, March 20, after the results were all compiled and studied, we met with Dr. McClain to establish the roadmap for treatment. We had some questions and concerns about the protocol that Texas Children's was using and we wanted to explore any alternatives. Dr. McClain said he needed some time to review and research some of the things we had discussed, so we met again the following Tuesday. After great discussion and prayer, we compared available protocols and decided to follow a "Stanford V" protocol which had never been used at Texas Children's Hospital.

To cover our bases and make sure we had done our homework,

Mel called Dr. Michael Link, Pediatric Oncology Physician at Stanford and talked to him over the phone. As we understood it, Stanford and St. Jude's Hospitals were the main ones who have used and studied the Stanford V protocol. The continued research that is being done on this protocol has allowed their studies to provide them with information to tweak it to be a better, more precise treatment for Hodgkin's patients.

We wanted to talk to someone who was very familiar with the protocol, had seen it in action and confidently could claim the truth of the percentages of success (which were 90%). We were able to get through to him because our neighbor Georgiana, who lives across the street, mentioned that her husband Rob's sister is a physician at Stanford and she possibly could accumulate some additional information. This is soooo God... Ends up that she had just done foot surgery on Dr. Link's daughter and they were friends... so she made the initial call on our behalf... and we were able to get right through.

We are blessed that we knew the power of God before this storm hit... for we knew He was trustworthy and HE would not leave us in time of trouble... And He never did!

Praise God wherever you are and in whatever situation He has allowed you to be in for His Glory will shine through!

Molly WILL be protected and embraced as she walks through this storm... We all will! I would come to learn more about the strong character of this child through this battle than I ever would have imagined. For those of you who have teenage daughters... you, too, will think of your child and wonder how you would handle this jolt if it hit you. Being the mom is the greatest honor and the most precious gift that God could have given me. My hope is that the writings in these next few pages will offer you an anchor to keep you steadied when something big blows through your lives... and that anchor is the Lord Jesus Christ.

The following e-mail represents the beginning of our journey. It was sent by one of my dear friends the day of our initial appointment before we knew what was wrong She knows my heart and so many times, as a kindred spirit, can tap into my thoughts that fall way below the surface.

I printed this out and kept it with me, pasted in the front of my notebook, throughout our journey. Many times I would refer back to it because, as you will read, it gave me a tremendous comfort and encouragement reminding me that God is "taking care of this."

To: Cathy
From: Jan G
Sent: Monday, March 13

My sweetest friend and sister in Christ…God has been talking to me ever since our time on the phone together this afternoon. He wanted me to share the following with you sooooo here goes: "My child, always, always, ALWAYS remember that this battle is NOT yours. I am your Abba Father and I will go before you in this journey and I will move the mountain. I have been with you all along and I will remain at your side. Fear not, for I am always with you. Before the thought is even formed in your spirit, I know what your need is and I will meet you at the very core of it. Molly is my child…she IS a King's Kid! I know the end from the beginning and all the in between. I will guide you and direct you in every decision made on her behalf. Be anxious for nothing, but through prayer and supplication just let go and let ME. The peace that passes all understanding will flow through you like a river. Be confident in this, that the good work I began in Molly, I will perform it until the day of Jesus Christ, my son. Let not your heart be troubled, neither let it be afraid. Be of good courage and I will strengthen your heart. Do not, do not, do not let the strongman get a foothold of fear within you. Take every thought of fear and anxiety captive to the glory of Jesus Christ. Know this; I will supply ALL your needs according to my riches in the glory of Christ Jesus. Remember, I have not given you a spirit of fear, but of power, and of love, and of a sound mind!"

Cathy, I love you so very much and hold you in my heart and in my prayers. Praise be to God from whom all blessings flow.

In His love,
Jan

To: Molly
From: Mom
Sent: Tuesday, March 21 (a week after the initial diagnosis)

Molly, I sat in the garage on an igloo last Monday after I had gotten home from being with you at the Doctor. It was the only place to just get away and hide and cry and tell God all the thoughts that were whirling around in my head. You were back at school. This was the beginning, the first CT. I had taken my phone with me because I was expecting a call from Dr. Muntz. Jan G. is the friend that God nudged to call me while I was out there. (She was God's reply to my cry for help). The above e-mail dated March 13, the day we found out the diagnosis, is what God put on her heart after we talked that afternoon. Molly, I know it sounds strange but she thinks and talks and experiences things a lot like I do.

Please keep this e-mail and read this prayer often.

I love you my dear Molly,
Mom

Praise God wherever you are and whatever situation He has allowed you to be in...His Glory will shine through!

[I have taught a bible study group for several years...and many of the friends whose responses you will read have been a part of that bible study somewhere along the way. These ladies are dear friends and many of us have met together for many years and studied God's word.

Kitty, the one who took this ball and rolled it was one of them, Jan; the one who sent the initial encouraging e-mail was another.

Most of the e-mails that are included are from these precious friends…and some are from friends who go way back before marriage or children, others are friends and families we have raised our children with and traveled with, and still others are friends who have graced our life's with their friendship when our paths have crossed through church, or organizations or committees or friends of friends or somewhere else. Wherever our paths crossed…It was God's hand that guided our friendships…and each was a designated PRAYER WARRIOR who God chose to be part of our lives. God has used each of them to serve as his loving hands on Earth. They were the wind that God sent to help us sail through this. They did their job well!]

To: Monday Bible Study Group
From: Cathy
Sent: March 20

Good Morning, Ladies:

We do have a diagnosis. Cancer: Hodgkin's Lymphoma, Phase IV. We have an appointment with Dr. McClain this morning to consider which road map to use for this journey.

SHE WILL BE HEALED!

There is no question. No question in our minds. God is clear on that!

Two stories for today:

This first story is about a dream I had on either Monday or Tuesday night; the days are running together. It was short, very concise, and very precise, but it was a dream I knew I was to remember:

I was standing alone…very calm…nothing in the background…CALM, CALM…a hand comes from my left and gives me a rolled up document…simply said: "This is your diagnosis!" I again calmly, no emotions said, "Thank you."

Another figure in a brilliant robe appeared on the right and extended his hand, gently took the document and said, "I'LL TAKE CARE OF THIS." And, that is who I have left it with. It is no longer something I have to hold. It is in God's hand!

Though there will be tears and fears, I will help Molly to find God's blessings each day…we all will.

The Second story is about the way that God works and His promise to go before us in the face of a storm.

Note: Lynda and David Tauber (the T's) have a 19 year old daughter named Rebekah who has been down this cancer road… Her diagnosis was different than Molly's; she has a cancer called Rabdiomysarcoma. It is a strong, resilient cancer which continues to reclaim territory in Rebekah's neck and head area. The drugs have not been able to defeat this monster of a disease in this precious child… but Rebekah is a warrior, the whole family is, and our mighty God has equipped them with His strength and His courage as they take on each day one at a time.

Shawn D. and I have been friends for many years. Leigh, Shawn's daughter and Molly have been friends since they were little and we have carpooled throughout high school. These were the friends we were with on Spring Break when Molly first showed the lump on her neck to her dad, Mel.

We had been back from vacation for a week and when I told Shawn on Friday that Molly had cancer… her first comment was "You should talk to the T's!".

Mel said Thursday someone had come to his office and asked, "Have you talked to the T's?"

Saturday morning Mel and I talked about when the best time to call the T's would be.

We went on an early walk and stopped for a visit with Dale H., our neighbor on the next street. He knew something was going on because his wife Carolyn had told him that she had seen me on a walk that week and she knew I was saddened about something. When we told him of Molly's diagnosis and what we were struggling with, he said he has been on an e-mail prayer list for Rebekah T. The e-mails have really been a great encouragement to him… maybe talking to the T's would help you.

The T's are friends from way back. Mel and David T. work in the same building and their paths often cross through business. No matter how long it had been since we had seen them, we could always pick up where we left off… but we would find that God would strengthen our friendship through events we could never have imagined. It will show how God goes before you and makes ready your path.

We had been invited to go to a wedding Saturday night. It was a small group of folks at the Rainbow Lodge. Cliff, an associate who Mel works with and a dear friend to both of us, was getting married to Angela, who we have grown to love as well.

There were just a handful of people we knew, most of them were from Mel's office. Our friends were concerned, as they had heard our news, and offered help in every way but talking about it was hard. I remember Sandra I. asking what protocol we would be on. (I didn't even know what "protocol" was.) She has a granddaughter who had leukemia at a very young age and she had spent a lot of time at Texas Children's Hospital in their Oncology Department. I remember her telling me to not be afraid to ask questions. We were still absorbing the jolt. And as far as what we needed and what we were in for, we had no idea. (This was the Saturday following the Monday when we found out the diagnosis.)

I had just gotten up from the table, Mel had left a few minutes earlier to speak to Cliff when there was a tap on my shoulder. It was Lynda T. Mel had seen David (her husband) and her walk in and briefed them about Molly. All I could say when I saw her was, "I need you."

She said, "How did I not know this for the whole week?" We stood in a corner of the room and talked for 30 minutes. It was like no one else was in the room. This was who God had sent to calm my heart. She gave me a "grocery list" of what to do and what to expect. Ex: How to work with the school, what to take with you to treatments, hang out in the Psalms, read David Jeremiah's Book, "A Bend in the Road", don't worry about calling people, they understand, it's okay to move a bed in your room to have her close (we never had to do that but we did try a monitor for a while…but even that ended up not being necessary) only take one day at a time, treatments don't hurt, etc.

God has gone before us. He knows the difficulty of this journey, but He is faithful.

When asked of David T., "What is the greatest thing you have learned?" His reply: "To take only this day, for God will give you what you need for THIS DAY"! When asked of Lynda T., she stood quietly thinking for a minute and said, "How much God loves us."

That no matter what we imagine, it still would only be a tiny grain compared to his abundant, abounding love.

She said you and Molly and your family WILL NEVER BE THE SAME AND YOU WILL PRAISE GOD for he has given you the honor of being his messenger!

The T's invited us for dinner on the following Wednesday, March 22nd. This time we had the pleasure of meeting Rebekah T. (We had only met her once years ago when she was little.) What a darling girl and so personable. She sat right there with Lynda and David and answered questions with poise and grace. Many of our fears were put to rest and after dinner we felt like they had taken the chill out of an unknown experience yet to come.

The rest of the week was pretty normal. Molly hung out with friends on Friday and Saturday, church on Sunday. My brother Tommy and his family came over and brought lunch. They had just gotten back in town from spring break and Molly and his girls Claire and Julie are all about the same age... and are good friends. They had missed each other. It was a fun time... and things seem to be normal even if it was for just a while.

John Crimmins, our Pastor and dear friend from Christ Evangelical Presbyterian Church came over Sunday late afternoon and prayed with our family. He pondered what Molly must be feeling knowing that tomorrow, Monday, March 27, she would begin her journey. The Lord put Isaiah 43:1–6 (NIV) on his heart about being scared. It's a wonderful verse to recall if fear had creped in; Molly remained calm... please Lord may I!

Israel's Only Savior

> 1. But now, this is what the LORD says—
> he who created you, O Jacob,
> he who formed you, O Israel:
> "Fear not, for I have redeemed you;
> I have summoned you by name; you are mine."

2. When you pass through the waters,
    I will be with you; and when you pass through
    the rivers, they will not sweep over you. When
    you walk through the fire,
      you will not be burned; the flames will not
    set you ablaze.
3. For I am the LORD, your God,
    the Holy One of Israel, your Savior;
    I give Egypt for your ransom,
    Cush [a] and Seba in your stead.

4. Since you are precious and honored in my
    sight, and because I love you,
    I will give men in exchange for you,
    and people in exchange for your life.

5. Do not be afraid, for I am with you;
    I will bring your children from the east
    and gather you from the west.

6. I will say to the north, 'Give them up!'
    and to the south, 'Do not hold them back.'
    Bring my sons from afar and my daughters
    from the ends of the earth.

This is the quote Shelley J. gave me the Monday we had our comprehensive diagnosis:

> There is nothing—no circumstance, no trouble, no testing—that can ever touch me until; first of all it has gone past God and past Christ, right through to me. If it has come that far, it has come with a great purpose, which I may not understand at the moment. But as I refuse to become panicky, as I lift up my eyes to Him and accept it as coming from the throne of God for some great purpose of blessing to my own heart, no sorrow will ever disturb me, no trial will ever disarm me, no circumstance

will cause me to fret, for I shall rest in the joy of what my Lord is!—That is the rest of victory."

Alan Redpat

To: Bible Study Group
From: Cathy
Sent: Wednesday, March 23
Subject: Continue meeting at my house

I don't know when I'll be back. We start chemo next Monday, but it gives me great joy for all of you to meet at my house. This is not an "I'm Sorry" deal!

How can you be sorry when the ALMGHTY GOD has chosen to MOLD you in a great way?! By Great Adversity!
BE WATCHFUL FOR HIS HAND IN YOUR LIFE.

Cathy

Praise God wherever you are and whatever situation He has allowed you to be in...His glory will shine through!

Phase I: The Battle Begins

Our First week of treatment... March 27. We were anxious; for this was the beginning and we really weren't sure of what to expect. New faces, new procedures, new place... new battleground.

To: Kitty
From: Cathy
Sent: Monday, March 27
Subject: GOD IS FAITHFUL

GOD IS SO FAITHFUL! Today went the best that it could go. Molly's stomach was a little iffy but she rallied. She has so much courage; oh, how I admire her. A journey just seems so long when you first begin it! She had a PICC line put in her arm this morning that will stay the duration of treatments (5 months). Jennifer needed to have a vision in her mind of where Molly would be. Of course we hadn't even thought of lunch and she trucked on down to the hospital on the rail from her downtown office and brought us all turkey sandwiches. Good thing too, because Molly was starved. We all were. Jennifer didn't stay the whole time but just enough to see the way that things worked and to meet Dr. McClain and document this first day.

This was the beginning of her treatments, and it was a relief that there was no pain... it just took time. We got home about 3:30 that afternoon. She was tired. It was a big first day!

NOTE: Texas Children's Hospital is just wonderful; their staff is professional and kind hearted, attentive... And no matter how busy they are they always were patient with who ever they were working with. The room is a big, colorful room that has several sections with seating arrangements from rocking chairs to couches. VCR's with videos going, most often cartoons or PG movies and children playing with assorted toys at play stations with tables and chairs to fit them. There was a bunch of activity and even a small kitchen providing water, tea, and snacks for families spending hours at their facility. It was the cheeriest place you could be as a pediatric cancer patient... and it had many distractions so you were not always focused on treatments.

They gave Molly 2 meds for nausea that have worked like a dream thus far. She even wanted a Baskin Robbins when she got home and we were well prepared. My friend Kristy had filled the fridge with a large container from BR with all different flavors so as to accommodate the whims that Molly might have. Thank you, thank you, thank you for your prayers! God is Listening to our requests! Praise Him... Please, praise Him and recognize His answer for today.

For one day at a time is all we are standing on and today has been a reflection of His grace. We were all pretty anxious; we now know the place where we will be, the faces of the nurses who will be treating her, and the protocol we will follow. Many of the unknowns have been addressed.

Note: We are on a roadmap of 12 weekly treatments; each Monday and an additional every third Tuesday. Dr. McClain says that this looks like a straight line but according to blood counts and platelets, it might vary a week and might have to be postponed. I remember rounding the corner of the reception desk at the Texas Children's Oncology floor when he said that and I thought: God is bigger than the routine odds.

THE PRAYER: MAY GOD SHOW THEM A STRAIGHT LINE IN MOLLY! NEW TREATMENT, BIG GOD.

Love you,
Cathy

P.S. Kitty, I am so sorry about the death of your precious friend Laurie. I know she was my friend too, but Kitty, you all were great friends and I love knowing how much you talked and each valued and shared your friendship. She will be missed by many and I know especially by you.

Praise God wherever you are and whatever situation He has allowed you to be in... His glory will shine through!

To: Kitty
From: Cathy
Sent: Tuesday, March 28
Subject: Focus on GOD

Okay, this is God's lesson; given to me on Tuesday, during a most remarkable quiet time! STAY FOCUSED... ON ME! He knows I am visual and it was like a poster!

1) Respect Me 2) Respect My Position 3) Respect my choices

Okay God, what is the difference between "who you are" and "what you do..."

> I AM !
> I AM the God of Love
> I AM the God of Hope
> I AM the God of Mercy
> I AM the God of Grace
> I AM the God of Forgiveness
> I AM the God of Strength
> I AM HOLY
> MY POSITION!
> This is what I do!
> I Heal—I am the Great Physician
> I Provide—I know your needs
> I Run the Universe—I am in control
> I Fight—the battles are Mine
> I Hear—and answer prayers
> I Comfort—when pain is near

I Strengthen—when you are weary
And then He gave me thoughts on CHOICE

Regarding God's choices:
1) They are not easy
2) They are not comfortable
3) They are not YOUR choice

My (God's) choice is to allow diversions in your life to show I will be victorious!

It is YOUR CHOICE to:
1) Be blown by the winds of fear or
2) Stand firm and trust Me, a rock which will never falter.

If we FOCUS on God, I mean really focus on God, then fear will grow strangely dim and lose its power to shake our bearings.

Our choice is how to react. . Do I accept
1) THE POWER OF THE ALMIGHTY GOD or
2) The power of fear?

Agree with God. Be at peace. Job 22:21 (NIV) "Submit to God and be at peace with him; in this way prosperity will come to you."

Yesterday, Molly had a procedure that we had to leave the room for, (this was the first time other than the initial surgery that she was alone). She had to get this PICC line in her arm. This PICC line would be the vehicle where all drugs would be administered. She would keep this in her arm for the duration of her treatments and it would alleviate her having to be stuck each time she had to have a blood check or receive treatments. She would always wear something with sleeves and no one ever even knew it was there. Each night we would have to flush the lines at home to keep them from getting clogged. It didn't hurt; we just had to remember to do it!

I had taken the verses that you left me last week and looked them up in my bible and read the commentaries on each of them. What power there is in God's word...! Thank you!

Love you,
Cathy

Praise God wherever you are and whatever situation He has allowed you to be in...His glory will shine through!

To: Kitty
From: Cathy
Sent: Thursday, March 30

Apparently—all these drugs have accumulated and the intense fighting has begun; war on the inside is reflected by total fatigue on the outside. Yesterday was tough. Now she needs strength. Man, this changes so quickly! The Dr. said this is the way it will be off and on. Some days better than others. I bet today is going to be a good one. The tutor comes and she is thinking about school stuff and her mind is preoccupied!

Love you,
Cathy

Praise God wherever you are and whatever situation He has allowed you to be in...His glory will shine through!

To: Cathy
From: Kitty
Sent: Thursday, March 30

Philippians 4:13 (NIV)
 I can do everything through him who gives me strength. *Molly can do all things including taking this strong drug through Christ who strengthens her.*

Exodus 15:2 The LORD is my strength and my song; he has become my salvation. He is my God, and I will praise him, my father's God, and I will exalt him. *We praise you, Lord, that You are Molly's strength.*

2 Samuel 22:33 It is God who arms me with strength and makes my way perfect.

2 Samuel 22:40 You armed me with strength for battle; you made my adversaries bow at my feet. *Thank you, Lord that you arm Molly with strength and she is armed for battle.*

Psalm 28:7 The LORD is my strength and my shield; my heart trusts in him, and I am helped. My heart leaps for joy and I will give thanks to him in song.

Psalm 29:11 The LORD gives strength to his people; the LORD blesses his people with peace.

Proverbs 31:25 She is clothed with strength and dignity; she can laugh at the days to come. *I love this one. Molly is clothed with strength and dignity and we will laugh with her as you see her through these days to come.*

2 Timothy 4:17 But the Lord stood at my side and gave me strength, so that through me the message might be fully proclaimed and all the Gentiles might hear it. And I was delivered from the lion's mouth. *What an awesome God who stands besides Molly to give her strength so she will be a witness to Your mighty work in her.*

Kitty

[Many of these e-mails are from Helene, JoAnn and Claudia. These are my friends and are the couples who Mel and I have traveled with and been friends with for many years. We have shared many seasons of life together; watching children grow up... sharing sorrows through death, and joys of captured memories. This jolt with Molly hit them pretty hard too... for they have known Molly and loved her since she was a baby.]

To: Cathy
From: Helene
Sent: Thursday, March 30

I just read and cried through your email to Kitty. I am in prayer for you and Mel and Molly and your entire family, constantly. Thanks be to God that you have such faith that you can allow Him to comfort you and that you are able to rest in His mighty strength!

I was thinking about my children and praying about some things in their lives I wanted God to be in control of and suddenly I stopped and thought about Molly. What really struck me was the way Mel always prays ..."You are a STRONG GOD." I thought about how we know that God is all powerful and everywhere, but when I began thinking about Molly and how BIG my prayers were about her and how comparatively insignificant the other things I was talking to God about seemed, I suddenly realized... that God is STRONG enough to handle everything for all of us. He knows our needs before we are even aware of them.

He knows exactly what is going on in your lives at this moment and tomorrow and next week... And He knows exactly what to do about each and every detail. As you said, He loves Molly even more than you and Mel do... He created her and trusted you to raise her up, to know Him and love Him..

Helene

To: Kitty
From: Cathy
Sent: Friday, March 31
Subject: Don't Hide the Story

Kitty, one thing I am learning is that I can't hide this story under a bushel; for it is God's story to do as He pleases. I appreciate you taking the initiative to help others be informed. Make this list as long as you like. From the outside looking in, this story is horrible and it is, BUT God knows He will conquer this disease and as Lynda T. wrote in an e-mail today "It is a journey." God's grace is being poured unto our family, especially Molly. She is courageous and sweet and so appreciative of the love that is being shown to her. She has been lifted so by prayers and notes and little surprises left at the door. I too am so grateful for the support.

This morning I asked God to give me something to chew on today and He put the relationship of He and His son on my heart. God watched His Son go through such pain and He must have been so pained by the vision, yet God knew the outcome. He knew that people would benefit from watching and loving and believing.

Oh, if Mel or I could step into her shoes... but our job is to uplift her and to help her care for her body the best that we are able. God knows the outcome. He understands our pain as we watch her battle this disease. He has been there... in his case He watched torture!

Last week God put on my heart the words: "How much do you love me? Do you love me as Peter did and will you deny me or do you love me with a faithfulness and trust that I AM RIGHT BESIDE YOU and through all of this I will be glorified?" Those are the questions that I not only have to answer but have to live. I know there will be tough days ahead, and I will cry, but God will be crying with me. Just look, we already are a week down! A few minutes ago Molly said, "Mom, this thing in my neck has almost gone." Her body is responding already, so we're here to hang on while God does the fighting. Remember when Shelley H said "I knew you all were praying for our family but I didn't know how much until you stopped?"

Note: Shelley's precious son Hamilton died in 2004. He was 23 years old. I wanted to know what he was like and when I asked Shelley to describe him this is what she said,

"I started thinking of adjectives and there were so many (as with any child), so I emailed both of my daughters to ask them. The adjectives that were common to all three of lists were; Hamilton was very kind, sensitive, funny and loyal." I didn't know Hamilton or even his family at that time. I only knew the extended family and the grandparents; they were members of our church. We were all praying for the peace and comfort of this family.

In 2006, Shelley came to my house for the first time for bible study. I think maybe Gina invited her. When I answered the door she introduced herself and I told her at that time that I was glad to finally meet her because I had prayed for her family. I said, "Do you know how many people were lifting you up in prayer that you hadn't even ever met?

She said "Yes, I knew that they were a lot of people praying for my family but didn't know how much until they stopped." It was a comment I will forever remember.

YES, WE FEEL YOUR PRAYERS. THANK YOU DEARLY!

If I don't get back to this e-mail—we will have chemo again on Monday am.

I have asked for prayers to protect Molly from fear—it is amazing how she has been shielded. Praise God.

Now she needs strength—for her body is so tired!

I Love you,
Cathy

Praise God wherever you are and whatever situation He has allowed you to be in... His glory will shine through!

To: Cathy
From: Helene
Sent: Sunday, April 2

It's Sunday night and tomorrow is chemo #2. I have been thinking of you and Mel and Molly all day. I have enjoyed Kitty's emails. It sounds like God has you safely tucked under His wing and that you are pretty comfortable there. There is something so very comforting about knowing that God is IN CHARGE. It takes all the worry about trying to decide what to pray for-what "you" want to happen. It is wonderful to realize that God knows what is going to happen. He is satisfied with the outcome because he knows all the good and the growth that will come out of it. If God is satisfied, we can be at peace and that is a very good place to be.

Helene

[Week two of treatments...April 3...we are starting to get in a routine. There are three different parts of the chemo treatment. This is the second; the third will be a two day. The girls (Jennifer and Jamie) check in all the time. They want to ask questions and want her to talk but when she is finished with treatments...she is finished...there is no taking about it! But she knows they are there! Each time, after a treatment, Mel would take Molly and me out for lunch to change the focus of the morning. Sometimes Jennifer or Jamie would join us...but Molly didn't want anyone else. She seemed to be okay for a few hours after and then she would crash late afternoon.]

To: Kitty
From: Cathy
Sent: Monday, April 03
Subject: The Notes Help

Kitty, you don't know how important these little notes are. Last night neither Molly nor I could sleep. She is taking this prednisone drug and it seems to get her and keep her very focused. She was doing math homework at midnight and at 12:30 organizing cosmetics. I, meantime, was diving into scripture. Lynda was right when she said hang out in the Psalms: Psalm 57 Be merciful to Molly...she will take refuge until these devastating storms pass; we all will. I will not be shaken! Psalm 62: in the shadow of my wings you will sing for joy, Psalm 63: Blessed is the Lord who DAILY bears us up, Psalm 63:19, Psalm 71: Be to me a rock of refuge, a STRONG FORTRESS, Psalm 71: I will deliver, Psalm 91 : 9–16, Psalm 103: who heals all of your diseases, and finally Psalm 127: HE gives sleep to his beloved...

After Molly had decided what she would wear if she is up to going to the tennis tournament, she called it a night. I sat next to her on her bed, rubbed her arm and she finally relaxed about 1:00 am. She was able to fall asleep. God had gotten us through another day. I had a few confessions to make about loving others conditionally instead of unconditionally! Sometimes I feel my nerves getting a little frayed... new challenges are okay, but there are just a bunch of them and when I add my emotions too! Well... God is trying to help me to see others through his loving eyes rather through my judging eyes. You would think among all this "REAL," "Hit the fan stuff" that these petty thoughts would be gone; but NO, there is still lots to clean in this heart of mine! If only I would or I could truly focus ALL of me on God. Oswald Chambers in "My Utmost for His Highest" got me the last couple of days!

Okay, here we are... another new day! Well, I am going to make Molly some breakfast!

Cathy

Praise God wherever you are and whatever situation He has allowed you to be in... His glory will shine through!

To: Kitty
From: Cathy
Sent: Monday, April 03
Subject: Molly's Prayer Warriors

Two down! We have figured out that we will have 12 treatments, 12 Mondays in a row, 2 are done. The first was intense. The even numbers 2, 4, 6, 8, 10, 12 will be easier weeks; 1, 3, 5, 7, 9, 11 will be the hard ones with intense treatment. We are counting backwards! Two are done, 12 and 11, 10 will be a combination of two days; Monday and Tuesday. Then we will be in single digits.

Today went well, her counts are good and the once noticeable spot on her neck HAS significantly diminished. This means that her body is responding well and that other effected cancer areas are also being broken up and destroyed. She will have radiation after the 12 chemo treatments.

We are trying to get her to focus on other things and this week she is hoping to feel good enough to go to some of the matches at the tennis tournament. You can't believe how terrific she is handling this. She takes one day at a time. Patiently waits for whatever anyone tells her to do, does it and then moves on. She is a calm soul and somehow her personality has allowed her to remain unruffled. She only wants information she needs to know and does not want a bunch of details. I think Mel and I have enough details for all of us. I thank you, thank you, thank you for your prayers. God is so very faithful.

Many have so graciously asked to do something, anything for us. We appreciate your thoughtfulness so much but really for right now, we are doing just fine. Mondays are big days and the last two Mondays when we have gotten home there have been notes for her at the front door. If you want to do something send a FUNNY note or a Way to go note or a congratulations, another one down note that would be great.

Kitty, thank you again for taking this on and forwarding these e-mails. It saves me so much time and helps to keep those who are sweet enough to be thinking about us informed.

Love,
Cathy

Praise God wherever you are and whatever situation He has allowed you to be in... His glory will shine through!

To: Cathy
From: Kitty
Sent: Monday, April 3

Thank you, Lord that Molly's sickness is not unto death, but to the glory of God. John 11:4 Praise you, Jehovah Raphe, that you are the Lord that healeth Molly. Exodus 15:26 Thank you, Lord, that healing is already being evidenced in Week 11!

Kitty

To: Kathy
From: Claudia
Sent: Monday, April 3

I think about you everyday!

Love,
Claudia

[Claudia had a trip planned and had to leave right after we found out about Molly. It was hard for us to communicate. We were just working through this day by day. Each figuring out what we can do. Molly stayed very reserved... and we all tried to maintain a positive attitude.]

To: Cathy
From: Kitty
Sent: Friday, April 7

Thank you, Lord, that Cathy, Mel, Molly and the entire family will demolish arguments and every pretension that sets itself up against the knowledge of God, and they take captive every thought to make it obedient to Christ. (2 Cor. 10:5) Father God, replace their anxious thoughts with Your thoughts. How great are your works, O LORD, how profound your thoughts! Psalm 92:4–6 Father, in the Mighty Name of Jesus, we bind the spirit of fear and we lose the spirit of peace in the hearts and minds of the Jodeit family. Guard their hearts and minds, Lord. We claim Psalm 91 for them that they will dwell in the secret place of the most High and abide under the shadow of the Almighty. Thank you Lord, that you are their refuge and their fortress: their God, in Him they will trust. They will not be afraid of the terrors of the night. Give Your angels charge over them, to keep them in all Your ways. Thank you that You deliver them from the spirit of fear and that You set them on high because they know Your name. With long life will You satisfy Molly and show her Your salvation. May they rest, Lord, knowing the battle is Yours. Grant them sleep for they know that the King of Kings and Lord or Lords has everything in His control.

In the precious, holy, healing Name of Our Lord and Savior, Jesus Christ.

Amen

To: Cathy
From: Claudia
Sent: Friday, April 7

Molly, How is it going? I tried to email you in Melbourne but it came back, probably a full mailbox. Hope you are still doing ok, I think of you everyday.

Love,
Claudia

To: Kitty
From: Cathy
Sent: Saturday, April 08
Subject: Prayers to pray for Molly

Kitty, I bought Molly a new Life Application Study Bible and I am highlighting these verses for her so someday when she goes to this book for wisdom she will be comforted by verses that have been prayed for her over this journey in her life. Lynda T. gave me a book called "A Bend in the Road" by David Jeremiah. It is a wonderful read if you are facing what he refers to as a "disruptive" moment in life. I am convinced that it is so important to fill, fill, fill your mind with good stuff all day; the Bible, Oswald Chambers, "My Utmost for His Highest," your e-mails, the David Jeremiah book, etc. because Satan so wants to take you to his dominion of fear and uncertainty. He wants, most of all, to replace the peace of God with his torment.

This is not just a battle with our family this is one that each of us faces everyday regarding something. I love the quote I once heard that said "take captive every thought and make it obedient to Christ."

I am anxious about next week. Molly has a new regiment of treatments and it will be Monday and Tuesday this week. Don't know what to expect but we have to be at the clinic for a much longer time. Mel is my earthly rock and reminds me that we will handle whatever is dealt... and in the words of Jennifer's friend Meredith... "Don't borrow trouble"...

Prayer Request:

Please pray that the blood work shows that her body is still healthy to ingest these coming treatments, that the meds for sickness work without pause, that God will continue to strengthen her in spite of the war she is buffeting, and that God's peace will encompass her from top to toe.

Lots of love to all of you, but I am especially grateful to God for His love, His faithfulness, and mighty presence in this battle.

Cathy

Praise God wherever you are and whatever situation He has allowed you to be in... His glory will shine through!

To: Cathy
From: Kitty
Sent: Saturday, April 8

Let the weak say, "I am strong!" (Joel 3:10) Thank you Lord that even though Molly may feel weak, she is strong in the Lord. Praise God, that You arm Molly with strength and make her way perfect. She will be ready for battle on Monday. (2 Samuel 22:33, 40)

Thank you, Lord, that Molly, whose hope in the LORD will renew her strength. She will soar on wings like eagles; she will run and not grow weary, she will walk and not be faint. (Isaiah 40:31)

And I pray that God's peace will encompass her from top to

toe, and the peace of God, which transcends all understanding, will guard Molly's heart and mind in Christ Jesus.

Cathy

To: Kitty
From: Cathy
Sent: Sunday, April 8
Subject: May you be blessed

(Philippians 4:7) Thank God for what he has done already and THANK HIM TOO FOR THE PLAN HE HAS FOR ALL OF THIS.

For somehow all who are involved with this child will be blessed and honored for going through this fire with her and with our whole our family. I thank God for each of you.

Cathy

Praise God wherever you are and whatever situation He has allowed you to be in... His glory will shine through!

To: Cathy
From: Cynthia
Sent: Sunday, April 8

Hey... I only know right now to say I love you deeply, and that God is holding your families lives in the palm of his hand. I'm standing beside you!

Love,
C

[My kindred spirit living in California... she knows how to cut right to the chase and has a sense of humor that goes on and on.

This is her serious side... she did stand right beside us from beginning till end]

To: Kitty
From: Lucy C
Sent: Sunday, April 8

Thank you, Kitty, for your kindness in sending me this email. We will continue praying and believing God for Molly's complete healing.

Love,
Lucy C

[This is a kneeling PRAYER WARRIOR... who I have been blessed to have by my side for many years. My children, all of them, have no idea the many times I have solicited the prayers on their behalf from this precious lady.]

[Week 3 of Treatments... M o n d a y, April 10 She is just trucking through this! Jennifer is trying to help her on her resume... and there is a home tutor to help her stay caught up in school. Distractions are good. Some friends gave her a couple of CD's having season episodes of her favorite shows. The outpouring of precious gifts and notes has been unbelievable. Molly's room has flowers that smell just wonderful. You don't think much about smells, but they are important.]

To: Kitty
From: Cathy
Sent: Monday, April 10
Subject: Molly

Kitty, what a blessing today has been. We got a great report for Molly from Dr. McClain. Blood cells, platelets, everything is in good shape and improvements over the whole body have been made just in this short time. She is called a rapid responder vs. a slow responder. The treatment today was our longest one yet and there was a standby nurse throughout the entire procedure in case there was a severe allergic reaction. NONE. Now we have gone through one of each of the regiments, the treatments from now on will be repeats of what has already been done. We are one fourth of the way through and you can tell Molly was glad for the report. It made these last couple of weeks worth the effort. She continues to be a wonderful sport; laid back, sense of humor in tact, very private about her thoughts, and seemingly confident that "it is what it is!" (A favorite quote from Wilhelmina, my precious friend and second mom who is married to my dad) This week there are no specific prayer requests rather Praises; for God has been faithful to "Take care of this." He is healing her body and protecting her from fear and has given wisdom to her care providers just as requested. So, just praise God—no "Pleases" just praises. Thank you for your constant support.

With love and appreciation,
Cathy

Praise God where ever you are and whatever situation He has allowed you to be in... His glory will shine through!

To: Cathy
From: Dawn
Sent: Tuesday, April 11

I just read your good Molly report from yesterday (Monday, April 10th), and I am so very happy that the treatments are going so well. God is so good. Remember that we are praying for Molly and for your family. Her quick response to treatment is surely the result of so very many prayers by so many loving family members and friends.

Love,
Dawn

[This is a friend Kitty introduced me to years ago who works in the same office with Kitty. We became fast friends when we both worked at the Redstone Building... she is such a sweetheart and dear friend.]

To: Cathy
From: Dana
Sent: Tuesday, April 11

Great news, so glad your day was so positive. This is one of my favorite bible verses is Psalm 91: 1–15 but this is starting at verse 9. If you make the Most High your dwelling-even the Lord, who is my refuge- Then no harm will befall you, No disaster will come near your tent. For he will command his angels concerning you to guard you in all your ways; "Because she loves me." says the Lord, "I will rescue her; I Will Protect her, for she acknowledges my name. She will call upon Me, and I will answer her; I Will be with her in trouble, I Will deliver her and honor her with long life, I Will satisfy her and show her my salvation."

With love and prayers,
Christine and Dana

[A friend and mom who has a daughter in Molly's class... she also is an adult Sunday school teacher at her church... I too love this verse]

To: Cathy
From: Kitty
Sent: Tuesday, April 11

Thank you, Jehovah Raphe, the Great Physician, Healer of Molly. We exalt You. Praise the LORD, O my soul: all my inmost being, praise His holy name. Praise the LORD, O my soul, and forget not all His benefits who forgives all Molly's sins and heals all her diseases, who redeems her life from the pit and crowns her with love and compassion, who satisfies Molly's desires with good things so that her youth is renewed like the eagle's Psalm 103:1–5 This is my favorite Psalm.

Kitty

To: Cathy
From: Susan K
Sent: Tuesday, April 11

Cathy, I just wanted to drop you a quick line to tell you that even though we don't know Molly, Larry and I are both praying for her and your family throughout this process. We loved the good report from Kitty today about her positive report. What a remarkable young lady. We have met all of your other children, so we have an idea of what a precious child she must be. You have such a tremendous faith and knowledge and it is something we can all learn from. We will pray praises this week for you all and wish you a very Happy Easter.

Much love,
Susan and Larry

[We met when we both had daughters at UT... and we still keep up through our daughters and mutual friends]

To: Cathy
From: Suzanne M
Sent: Tuesday, April 11

Bless the Lord, O my Soul and all that is within me... Bless His Holy Name! Continuing with you in prayer through this journey...

Love and Hugs,
Suzanne

[A strong friend in the Lord... and a wonderful bible study teacher]

To: Cathy
From: Jill
Sent: Tuesday, April 11

Cathy,
 "The Lord is good! He is a stronghold in times of trouble, and He knows those who trust in Him" Nahum 1:7 Charles and I are rejoicing over Molly's good reports. Praise, honor and glory to Him.

I love you,
Jill

To: Cathy
From: Kay S
Sent: Wednesday, April 12

I just want you to know you are being prayed for and you are in our thoughts every minute! You know I am here for you so USE ME.

Happy Easter and I love you,
Kay

[My sweet friend... in bible study for many years, she is a terrific listener as well as encourager]

From: Cathy
Sent: Sunday, April 16
To: Kitty
Subject: Molly's Week Nine Countdown Begins

Kitty, Molly and I were just talking about this whole treatment so far. She is really surprised that she has felt so good and been able to get out and do things with friends. This week is an even week, so it will be a shorter treatment session. What a blessing that she got to go to church and then to lunch with the family. Jennifer is getting a new puppy today and Molly is beside herself with excitement. So fun to see her happy. There is a lot to be said about what you think about, and how you tune your thoughts. It is kind of like a radio station, change the channel if you just start hearing a bunch of Blah, Blah, Blah, and find something to think about that lifts your spirits, and helps you to look at life in a joyful way. Philippians 4:8 (NIV) Finally, brothers, whatever is true, whatever is noble, whatever is right, whatever is pure, whatever is lovely, whatever is admirable—if anything is excellent or praiseworthy—think about such things.

Last week I started letting thoughts drift through my mind about the unknown, and boy did it get me. Then I realized that I needed to concentrate on TRUTH and FACT, and let all other anxious moments be pushed out. I was talking to Kitty about this and she reminded me that when we Praise and Worship God, our thoughts are strong and it is hard for Satan to compete with. (It is funny how God gives you a friend who says just we he knows will do your heart good… I needed Kitty to tell me this and I know God put the words in her mouth to speak them to me… at this time) So when my mind starts wandering, now I start praising, and remember who God is and what he has done… Though circumstances are changing all about me, I worship a God who never changes… He can't love me any more, and can't be any better or any wiser or any greater than he is NOW! It is on this that I try to stand without wavering!

We are counting down and are grateful for the progress that has already been made and look forward to finishing tomorrow—then we will be one fourth of the way through!

Thank you for your continued prayers—and love,
Cathy

> Romans 5:1–5 "Therefore since we have been justified through faith, we have peace with God. Through our

Lord Jesus Christ, through whom we have gained access by faith into this grace which we now stand.

Praise God wherever you are and whatever situation He has allowed you to be in... His glory will shine through!

To: Kitty
From: Cathy
Sent: Tuesday, April 18
Subject: Molly Gets a New Puppy

I am the Lord who heals Molly. Exodus 15:26

Another treatment down—we are a quarter of the way through the chemo—God has blessed us greatly—still good platelets, red-white blood cells in tact, all is going well.

Mel took Molly to pick out a new lab puppy today. There were six left in the litter. We met in Memorial Part and after just a few minutes Molly made her choice. She chose the sweetest pup, a lot of pep, not too wild, very affectionate and such a precious beautiful face. She was a yellow lab but her coloring was more of a white color. Molly is happy with her choice and has named her new lab Bentley, a name she has loved and has held on to since sixth grade. She knew the day would come when she could use it. Bentley would serve as a true companion during this battle... The day had come!

We go for a PET test this morning and a CT; we will have the results by week's end—they are expected to be favorable as the neck lymph nodes from the outside have disappeared. It really is amazing to see how God has already answered your prayers and ours. May God bless you and honor you for your intercessory prayers. Thank you again to so many of you who have sent specific verses using Molly's name; His glory is shining through!

Love,
Cathy

P.S. Specific prayer: Molly has a PICC line in her arm where the meds and chemo are introduced into her body; there is one line but it splits at the end into two parts; a short one and a little longer one. Yesterday one of them had clogged a little and it took a while to pressurize it and get it going. This was the first time we had had any difficulty. It is of the utmost importance that these lines stay working these next 8 weeks and that they don't need to be replaced… and that somehow her body will be able to differentiate between a foreign object vs. a necessary clean vessel for meds… and not come to the rescue with these little flurries that clog the lines!

Cathy

Praise God wherever you are and whatever situation He has allowed you to be in… His glory will shine through!

To: Cathy
From: Gina
Sent: Sunday, April 16

Prayer for Molly from Gina: "Therefore since we have been justified through faith, we have peace with God. Through our Lord Jesus Christ, through whom we have gained access by faith into this grace which we now stand. And we rejoice in the hope of the glory of God. Not only so, but we also rejoice in our sufferings. Because we know that suffering produces perseverance; perseverance, character and character, hope. And hope does not disappoint us because God has poured out His love into our hearts by the Holy Spirit whom He has given us. Romans 5:1–5!

Gina

[Spirit of compassion describes this tearful warrior… and bible study friend and great encourager]

[Week Four of treatments… April 17… countdown, one third of the way through. We are hanging in there.]

From: Cathy
Sent: Tuesday, April 18
To: Kitty
Subject: Additional Tests

We just got back from tests this morning, Molly is starved: Southwell's BLT was the crave. She hasn't eaten since dinner last night. This was the worst day she has had since she found out about this diagnosis. We had had each of these tests before, but one thing had changed since first look. After examining original tests closer they found that the initial cancer had spread throughout her body and was not only above the stomach but traces were in one of her lungs and her spleen.

We were told this a couple of weeks ago. They had seen it on the original pictures but after looking at the pictures more closely decided that this was an area that needed to be highlighted as well. We expected the tests that we had come to take were would be the same as the ones taken in earlier weeks. They were not! The exception was that the whole body would need to be scanned, not just the neck and chest area. This meant... that yuck tang stuff. Molly is not so good with surprises, and this was a big one. She has been the very best of sports on everything thus far but this was her limit. She is a light liquid girl anyway and this stuff was not only awful but there was a bunch of it. I know there are those of you reading this who know just what I am talking about.

I called Dr. McClain to see if it was an absolutely necessary test. After chemo yesterday, no food since dinner, and a stomach that was iffy, she was really sinking... Fast! He said, "Yes, it is necessary because we need good photos. Tell her to just TRY to get as much of it down as she can." He would do the best with the contrast shots that would be retrieved. After about 30 minutes her stomach was really shot. Molly did do the best she could. When we walked in they told her she would have to have an IV for the iodine. "Nope no IV" (I wasn't very diplomatic) One surprise was enough and this is why we have the PICC line. (Remember, she is scared of needles and an IV is not just a prick on the arm.) They fussed and talked and looked at the PICC line and finally made a decision to honor the request on Molly's behalf. The PICC line then was used as the vessel to administer the dye and she didn't have to be stuck.

You really do have to be an always thinking strong advocate for your child. For procedures are often just an "as is" way of doing things without true regard for the patient. Later I was asked if I was Irish; guess I was a little demanding! Oh well! This was my daughter and I will fight whatever meager battle I am given, mine are the small battles for her comfort, in comparison to the grand battles for health that she is fighting everyday. We all left on good terms but unfortunately they will remember us next time.

One thing I am learning through all of this is you have to be your child's advocate. Be smart, do your homework, ask questions, and think out of the box. You know your child and know how she best responds to situations. For Molly: No quick changes...if you give her time to absorb the situation and work through it in her mind...she is fine!

No one else is going to stand in her corner like you would as her parent. So many times the routine "way to do it" is standard and time has not been taken to rethink a situation for the comfort of the individual patient.

2 Chronicles 15:7 But you, take courage...Do not let your hands be weak, for your work shall be rewarded! They did get good pictures in spite of it all! And we were able to sidetrack the extra prick!

Bentley was perfectly timed...SHE was such a wonderful encouragement for Molly and gave her something to look forward to after a tough morning...nothing like a new puppy taking a nap with you on you bed.

We did have a chance to see the results of the PET test: God is awesome...the first image 4 weeks ago was covered with blotches over her whole body that signified cancer spots. Today you just can't believe how clear her body image was. The smudges were gone... the chemo has worked! What a blessing! God above all, Molly's youth and attitude, Dr. McClain, TCH professional staff, Stanford V protocol and loyal prayers of dear friends have all been factors in this success. We don't have results of the CT scan yet. It was explained to me that the PET scan was like the architecture of the body and the CT scan tells you what the people inside the building are doing. I love it when the explanation is on the bottom shelf and I can understand it!

I was sitting in the room while Molly was being scanned and thought," Why is it that when any of us hear the word cancer we cringe and get so anxious? Why was I so anxious? I guess because I have seen how precious friends have suffered and how dear friends and parents have died and because it is something that we really can't get our hands around." I thought about the word cancer and came up with this:

C.A.N.C.E.R.–"C"HRIST "A"LWAYS "N"EGOTIATES "C"IRCUMSTANCES for (His)"E"TERNAL "R"ICHES

Whatever the circumstances…health, relationships, finances, work, whatever; GOD is in charge, and the battle is HIS!

> 2 Chronicles 20:15, 20:17: We may not fight an enemy army, but every day we battle temptation, pressure and "rulers" of this present darkness who want to rebel against God.

Remember as believers, we have God's spirit in us. If we ask for God's help when we face struggles, God will fight for us and GOD ALWAYS TRIUMPHS.

How do we let God fight for us?
1) By realizing the battle is not ours, but God's
2) By recognizing human limitations and allowing God's strength to work through our fears and weaknesses
3) By making sure we are pursuing God's interests and not just our own selfish desires
4) By asking God to help us in our daily battles

So remember–CHRIST ALWAYS NEGOTIATES our CIRCUMSTANCES for His ETERNAL RICHES–(notice the our vs. his)
With Love and appreciation,
Cathy

Praise God wherever you are and whatever situation He has allowed you to be in...His glory will shine through!

To: Cathy
From: Audrey
Sent: Tuesday, April 18

Indeed, in our hearts we felt the sentence of death. But this happened that we might not rely on ourselves but on God, who raises the dead. He has delivered us from such a deadly peril, and he will deliver Molly. On Him we have set our hope that he will continue to deliver Molly, as you help us by your prayers. Then many will give thanks on our behalf for the gracious favor granted us in answer to the prayers of many. 2 Corinthians 1:9–11

Audrey

[A sweet bible study friend...and I loved the part of the verse at the end where it says, many would give thanks for the gracious favor God would grant through answered prayers...God is granting us favors for Molly each day]

To: Kitty
From: Cathy
Sent: Wednesday, April 19
Subject: Molly's results from PET and CT

Kitty, we just got a call from Dr. McClain who has looked at both the CT and the PET tests. He is beside himself. Totally amazed! He expected a good report but not this great of one. The word he used was EXTRADORDINARY! She has outdone anything he expected. This has been an encouraging experience for Molly as yesterday was the first time she had seen the first scan that showed the cancer all over her body. She gasped and almost started crying and then Cynthia, the sweet tech, who was the one who has gave Molly her first PET test and told us to ask TCH to leave in the IV, said, "Lets go take this test and I will bring you into the computer room and show you immediately the results. Forty five minutes later we saw the image… ALL was clear, except for one small hardly noticeable smudge on her neck. It is very small and it must have taken the expert eyes, we couldn't see it! Cynthia said to Molly, "See what you have been working on so hard this month?" It was such a visual to her and to all of us, a reality that prayers that have been answered.

It was verification that over these past days that she has tolerated the meds, the requirements, the maintenance of her PICC lines, the early mornings, the long waits, and the school thing and it had been worth it! The lymph nodes have shrunk 50% to 70%. Dr. McClain said, that too, is amazing in this length of time. These results will not change the protocol! Darn! We still have 8 weeks to go followed by radiation. Thank you, thank you thank you. Two appointments were cancelled for tomorrow because of these results. There are just blessings everywhere!

Prayer Request: Praise God, please, Praise God! Thank him for listening and answering our requests.

Psalm 105:1–3—O give thanks to the Lord, call on his name, and make known his deeds among the peoples. Sing to him, sing praises to him, and tell of his wonderful works. Glory in his holy name let the hearts of those who seek the Lord rejoice.

One more request: May God use this case to blaze a trail for new Hodgkin's patients to have as a possible alternative for treating this disease. This is the first time TCH has used the "Stanford V" protocol for treating Hodgkin's. Dr. McClain was courageous and willing to step out and try this alternative regime. It has been used by Stanford and St. Jude's and has proven to be 90% beneficial in curing Hodgkin's patients.

A note here about Dr. McClain, our oncology doc: We adore him and his gentle spirit. He is quite smart and well respected worldwide in the Oncology circles not to mention by us and his many patients and his staff. We are grateful for his integrity, ingenuity and his constant concern in honoring and conquering fears and apprehensions that Molly has had about hospitals and needles etc. He always went one step further to listen and work with us no matter what the concern was. He is truly our God sent Doctor.

Cathy

Praise God wherever you are and whatever situation He has allowed you to be in...His glory will shine through!

To: Cathy
From: Jan G
Sent: Wednesday, April 19

My heart rejoices in you Lord, for you are my strong shelter in times of trouble and stress, my hiding place to whom I may continually resort...my Father who lovingly provides for me...my Shepherd who guides and protects me...my Champion who upholds my cause as His child and defends me. I will rest in your love for you rejoice over me with shouts of joy. You act on my behalf, accomplishing what concerns me and fulfilling Your purpose for me as I call on You. I am filled with Your comfort as I take refuge in the shadow of Your wings! I love you girls!

Jan

[Whenever I would see her name on an e-mail I would know I was getting ready to read a note that would fill my heart with God's encouragement that I would need at that moment]

To: Cathy
From: Cynthia
Sent: Wednesday, April 19

My heart is full and grateful for this news and I praise God for his obvious hand in Molly's life! I'm celebrating this step with ya'll and continue to look to him for each step to come.
Open hands...right?! God cannot fill anything but open containers.

I love you,
C

[Notice the Ya'll and right?!... that will give you a hint into her personality]

To: Cathy
From: Mary Leslie
Sent: Wednesday, April 19

Hi Cathy! We are so happy and so thrilled for Molly! God is so good and so faithful... what a miracle that continues to unfold, not to mention the power of faith and hope that continues to be a part of Molly's ministry through this challenge. I know God continues to bless the lives of nurses, doctors and patients that meet all of you, not to mention old friends like me! Thank you for sharing your walk... and letting us pray for you. Our prayers now have so much praise and thanksgiving! I want to see this precious puppy! Have a good night.... our prayers continue.

Mary Leslie

[A long time friend... filled with great wisdom]

To: Cathy
From: Helene
Sent: Wednesday, April 19

I just read your "Kitty" email about Molly's test results. I can hardly type, I am crying so hard. "It's a Miracle" is just a phrase to a non-believer. It does not represent God's intervention or control of a problem. We know God has the power over life and death-over everything and everyone. He has chosen to use Molly and your precious family to demonstrate His mighty power. Praise, Praise, Praise! I also am so touched by what an advocate for Molly you are.

You challenged everything and everyone who wanted to do things that would trouble Molly. You challenged them and you showed Molly that you were there for her and that you would protect her and take care of her. God gave you the strength to stand in His stead for Molly.

As believers we are so lucky. We never need to face difficult situations alone. We always have our Heavenly Father by our side to take over for us. We can take comfort in knowing that the Creator of the Universe is by our side always. I am so very happy for you and Molly and your entire family. What wonderful news!

Love,
Helene

To: Cathy
From: Shelly H
Sent: Wednesday, April 19

Praise the Lord—what wonderful news!

Shelly

To: Cathy
From: Dave P
Sent: Wednesday, April 19

What AWESOME news! Thank you for making my week. Please keep me in your email group, as I will continue to forward and keep Molly's teachers informed. We all pray every day.

10th Grade Principal,
Dave

[This man turned somersaults for Molly...what a blessing he was throughout this entire process...not to mention wonderfully encouraging. He teared up when he was told about Molly's cancer and has a true heart of gold. He was the liaison between Molly all of her teachers and kept them posted as to her status.]

[The following is an e-mail is from my friend Lindy. But before you read it, I want you to know her story because it will help you understand the strength with which her words hit my heart. We have been friends for many, many years and she has gone through the cancer storm. She and her husband Larry celebrated her son's short life with unsurpassed grace. Lindy and Larry's son Bo died of liver cancer in 1985 at the age of 12. "Bo's Place" is named in loving memory of Laurence Bosworth "Bo" Neuhaus, Jr.

Bo's deep spiritual convictions, faith, humor and openness were strength to those who knew and loved him during his illness and following his death. "If I should die any time soon," he wrote, "I want balloons, a lot of helium balloons, and fireworks because I want it to be a celebration. God would want it that way and therefore, so do I."

Bo left behind a legacy of warmth and love. He also left behind a family who mourned their loss with a celebration of both balloons and tears. Through their experience, Bo and his family exemplified the spirit of hope, healing and growth, which was an inspiration in the development of a program in Houston "Bo's Place" for grieving children and their families.

"Bo's Place" offers a unique program that provides free grief support services to children and their families who have experienced the death of a parent or sibling.

Bo's Place is founded on the belief that children need to share with other grieving children in order to heal. Bo's Place offers the only ongoing program for grieving children and their families in the greater Houston area.]

To: Cathy
From: Lindy
Sent: Wednesday, April 19

Cathy,

I have wanted to write you and let you know that you and Molly and Mel are in our prayers daily. I just heard about Molly and am just so sorry she is having to go thru this ordeal, and being a mother, I can relate to everything you said in your email. (I stole your email address off of a forward that a friend sent to me. How proud and elated God must be in your faithfulness. You are right, it is God's battle, not ours, and His grace will shine thru it all. Please know that I am yours if you ever need to talk, cry, hit something, throw something, curse, anything you need. I have done it all. And please put me on your email list so I can keep up with Miss Molly. Please know that Larry and I care so much!

Love,
Lindy.

I am so thrilled for the good news. God's grace is immeasurable, that is for sure.

To: Cathy
From: Cynthia
Sent: Thursday, April 20

But they that wait upon the Lord shall renew their strength; they shall mount up with wings as eagles; they shall run, and not be weary; and they shall walk, and not faint. Isaiah 40:31
  The Lord your God is with Molly, he is mighty to save. He will take great delight in Molly, he will quiet Molly with his love, he will rejoice over Molly with singing. Zephaniah 3:17

How can we but love Him when we know that He

numbers the very hairs of our heads, marks our path, and orders our ways?—Charles Hadden Spurgeon

Cynthia

[I can see her sitting in the early morning drinking her tea as she has her quiet time with the Lord and then she shared it!]

To: Cathy
From: Beth
Sent: Thursday, April 20

Praise God from whom all blessings flow.

Beth

[A gentle spirited warrior and friend]

To: Cathy
From: Jill
Sent: Thursday, April 20

Cathy,
   I am overwhelmed with joy over these reports. Molly is indeed His personal concern and He is her personal bravery. My heart is full of praise for He is doing a great thing.

Sharing deeply in your joy with all my love,
Jill

To: Cathy
From: Sally
Sent: Thursday, April 20

Cathy,

I have been awed and reborn with every update on sweet Molly. He is indeed a God of impossibilities! Oh, how much He must love her! And how He must marvel at the love so many people have for his precious child! Her name must be forever before His throne—and how he has honored your faith through her miracles!

I am not sad when I picture you and Molly; I am filled with JOY! She is being rocked in her mother's loving arms and held in her Heavenly father's all powerful arms... and I marvel at the changes and the miracles happening in your lives minute by minute. I forever thank God for allowing me to share your faith and thank Him daily for what He has done in Molly's life today... and PRAISE Him for the gifts He will unwrap for you each and every day of this ordeal. OUR GOD IS INDEED A GOD OF MIRACLES AND IMPOSSIBLITIES.

Thank you, Lord, for what you are doing in Molly's life and may YOU receive ALL the Glory for the miracles you have bestowed daily on Molly! Take away her fears and doubts... and replace them with a peace that truly does passeth all human understanding.

I love you,
Sally

[This is one of my sweet friends from church... her family usually sits a few rows behind us... you know how you have your spot in church]

To: Cathy
From: Gina
Sent: Friday, April 21

We are so happy for you Molly...

Prayer is a fragrant dew, but we must pray with a pure heart to feel this dew. There flows from prayer a delicious sweetness, like the juice of very ripe grapes. Troubles melt away before a fervent prayer like snow before the sun... Prayer is the holy water that by its flow makes the plants of our good desires grow green and flourish, that cleanses our souls of their imperfections, and that quenches the thirst of passion in our hearts.
—John Vianney (1786—1859) French Priest

Love,
Gina Saour

[This is my green thumbed friend... notice the water and plants and fruits... her garden is literally filled with beauty and butterflies]

in reply to Gina's reply:

To: Cathy
From: Georgiana
Sent: Friday, April 21

Dear Cathy,

I thought you might be interested in the author of that last verse by John Vianney. He is also known as the Cure of Ares and is a great saint in the Catholic Church. Apparently, he was not considered smart enough for the priesthood and it took him a long time to get in. He had the gift of reading what was in people's hearts and they would line up way before dawn to have him hear their confessions. It was also said that Satan would physically attack him and beat him up. When he died, his body did not decay and you can still see it somewhere in France.

Love,
G

[my neighbor and front yard friend... many a night as I would walk through the house late when everything was dark and quiet and I could see her light was on and just knew that she was right there… just a call away]

The Fight Continues

Week five of treatments... April 24... Jenn and Jamie continue to try to encourage her. Molly really doesn't talk about this. So they have to go through me to get any updates or ideas as to what has been going on. Tom wants to know the facts... the logistics of the journey... and Mel, my sweet Mel comes home each day from work heavy hearted, yet knowing that we are doing all that can be done. We continue to see God's mighty hand and the improvements from the scans are a great encouragement.

To: Kitty
From: Cathy
Sent: Saturday, April 22
Subject: Molly week 5

Thank you for your continued prayers. We go in for the 5th treatment of 12 on Monday. These are the strongest 3 drugs. Please pray for Molly's body to continue to heal and that her body tolerates these drugs. Please don't stop praying because of the great report we had this week; it is through your prayers that God had honored your requests and we covet them and depend on them so.

Specific Prayers—Molly to have tolerance for drugs; continued healing; lymph nodes would continue to decrease in size; any hiding cancer cells would be revealed and killed; praise for the deeds God has already done; that the existing blotch on her PET Scan neck image would be healed and disappear.

Thank you for the many sweet e-mails and verses of encouragement and praise that so many of you sent last week. We serve a great God!

Cathy

Praise God wherever you are and whatever situation He has allowed you to be in... His glory will shine through!

To: Cathy
From: Jan G
Sent: Saturday, April 22

For my sweet friend and precious Molly: Thank you my gracious and sovereign God, that You have been with me and carried me from the day of my birth until today... that you have known my whole life, from beginning to end, since before I was born. Thank You that in your gracious plan to bless and use me, you've allowed me to go through hard times. I am so grateful that you're so good at reaching down and making something beautiful out of even the worst situations! Thank You for being my best friend, my wonderful counselor, my ever-present help; that you are available around the clock, seven days a week! Psalm 139:13–14, "For Thou did form my inward parts... I will give thanks to You for I am fearfully and wonderfully made."

I love you girls!
Jan

[When she prays out loud, it is truly like the Lord is standing right beside her... and he is, but she makes him so truly real you feel like you can reach out and tangibly touch him]

To: Molly
From: Gina
Sent: Tuesday, April 25

Let your roots grow down into Christ and draw up

nourishment from Him. See that you go on growing in the Lord and become strong and vigorous in the truth. Colossians 2:7

The words of the Lord are seeds sown in our hearts by the sewer. They have to fall into our hearts to grow. Meditation and prayer must water them and obedience keep them in the Light. Thus, they will bear fruit for the Lord's gathering.—George MacDonald

Dear Molly,

May you continue to improve and may you gain strength and feel comfort from the prayers of your friends and family.

Love,
Gina

[This marks the first month. We are still stepping through this journey one small step at a time. Molly was given a poster from the Young Life Sophomore girls. It has the numbers 1–12 (the # of treatments) on it in big calendar boxes. After each treatment we would mark the designated # out with big black X's. And on each Monday after treatment they would have a surprise waiting at the front door. Those were some of the little things that were perks for her day. They thought they were doing it for Molly... I was just as appreciative... for they gave me something to look forward to as well! What a precious group of girls to have gone to so much trouble and who would stay focused on that idea of generosity through the entire 12 treatments.]

To: Kitty
From: Cathy
Sent: Thursday, April 27
Subject: Tough Week for my Molly

We are now on Thursday of this week. Tough, tough week. The drugs this week are the most intense... But we only have to do this series 3 times and yesterday was the second, so only one more. Next week should be a little easier. What bugs us is that with such a great report last week you would think you would get to have a break. But it has been explained to us that the reason this protocol is so effective is that you don't break the cycle... and all those cells that are thinking about regenerating are going to be zapped. Apparently there are different phases of a cancer cell... the mature ones, the growing ones, and the planted ones. These signs are showing us the effect on the mature ones.

I often times think of God and the pain He must have felt when he was watching Christ going through the terrible torture that he did and knowing he was so innocent. I just look at Molly and think she is so innocent and only 16. I can't ask "Why?" Only "How" will God use this battle in HER life for HIS glory... and I think, This is HER story... no matter how much any of us are there to help or pray or love her... we can't be in her shoes... or feel what she feels... we can only support her!

I remember that story in the bible about Moses and the Israelites fighting the Amalakites; Exodus 17:11 As long as Moses' hands were held up, they were winning. But when he dropped his hands they started losing. That is kind of the way I look at it with Molly. It is her battle but she needs us all there to help her hold up her hands... she will win. This past month has gone really well. The drugs are working, the fears of all the new protocol have been faced; but these next 7 weeks of chemo present new challenges... she needs courage, strength, patience and CONFIDENCE!

Thank you my friends! Thank you for being concerned when you didn't get an e-mail: shows this system is working. We do not take for granted one minute your thoughts and prayers... for life is busy for everyone and each of you has your own battles and life sidelines that you are dealing with. This is big but your challenges are big too! Always remember, We worship an almighty God! I hope that you will not only go to God about this big stuff but also with your whole heart... and what you are struggling with in your lives. He is not only listening to you when you lift up a prayer for Molly; He wants to love you and guide you and comfort you too!

It is with love and true appreciation that I send this,
Cathy

Praise God wherever you are and whatever situation He has allowed you to be in... His glory will shine through!

To: Cathy
From: Jennifer
Sent: Thursday, April 27

Good job, Mom.

[The encouragement from my children touched my heart in a way they will never know... something as little as this e-mail]

To: Cathy
From: JoAnn
Sent: Thursday, April 27

Good morning my sweet friend,

Yes, I have so missed the updates on Molly so that I could know EXACTLY what to pray, although I keep her in my thoughts and prayers all day long anyway. Just reading your e-mail this morning made me feel as if I was right there by your side listening to your sweet voice of confidence and encouragement which you so beautifully exude through the HOLY SPIRIT and emit to everyone and right now particularly to precious Molly. What BLESSINGS you and Mel are right now to her and it is such a BLESSING that you have her all to yourself to do whatever she wants to do. Know that I am by your side "in spirit" as you are taking care of Molly and at the same time I feel your sweet "spirit of friendship" right next to me as I lift you all up in prayer.

In much love and prayer,
Jo ann

> The Lord is Molly's rock, her fortress and her deliverer; Molly's God is her rock, in whom she takes refuge. He is Molly's shield and the horn of her salvation, her STRONGHOLD. Psalm 18:2

To: Cathy
From: Gary and Grace
Sent: Thursday, April 27

Dearest Cathy,

You and your precious family have been on our minds and hearts and in our prayers continually. Thank you for your beautiful, hopeful words. I loved the scripture you brought to us through this; Moses with his hand held high. Lean on God and to think about all of us with all of our troubles when you are in the midst of the desert. We know that there will be dark days ahead, but what hope we have in God that indeed Molly's life in some way will bring glory to our Father. We can pray for healing, and for comfort and for peace, and put her, and you and yours in His hands.

We love you,
Grace, Gary and Carrie

[Wonderful dear college friends... Grace was a sorority sister and Gary was Mel's roommate... pretty sweet that they stayed with us through this]

To: Cathy
From: Brian and Leslie
Sent: Thursday, April 27

We had an e-mail forwarded to us about Molly and you are so right about her being in God's hands! I know what she and your family are going through right now is challenging but your faith speaks volumes and I know she will win! We just want you to know that your family and Molly are in our thoughts and prayers.

Love you guys,
Brian and Leslie

[Another long time friend from college... Brian and Gary and Mel all lived in the same apartment... Brian and Leslie just moved back from Dallas and live in the Woodlands... we don't have a chance to see them much but when we finally do we can just pick right up!]

To: Cathy
From: Jill
Sent: Thursday, April 27

How has Molly's week been? I am awaiting Kitty's update. God is performing a mighty miracle in and through Molly and the ramifications are staggering. My prayers continue to be ones of highest praise to Him for his mercy, power, might, and faithfulness. As you and Mel keep the umbrella of protection held high over your family, Charles and I and countless others count it a real privilege to be a part of this concert of prayer for your precious Molly. With much love in our Lord, in Whom we live, and move, and have our being, (Acts 17:28)

Jill

[Jill and her husband Charlie are dear church friends... God sent Jill to me as a mentor and friend years ago and I have cherished her wisdom and have watched her often from afar. I have taken mental notes on how to let GOD have the reigns of my life... she does it so gracefully and seemly without effort]

To: Kitty
From: Cathy
Sent: Friday, April 28
Subject: Molly's Umbrella

Have mercy on me, O God have mercy on me; for in You

> we take refuge, we will take refuge in the shadow of your wings until this storm has passed. Psalm 57:1

My sweet friend Jill e-mailed me today about Molly being under the protective umbrella of Mel and me. I had to laugh a minute because it brought back memories of several trips to New York where I had been with one of my girls and we had been caught in one of those thunderstorms. We would buy a cheap umbrella from the sidewalk vendor and within minutes the umbrella would be inside out and in a cone shape reaching towards the sky thus leaving us unprotected, wet and in absolute surrender to the storm at hand.

Have to admit that is kind of the way it has been this week—You know when you are in a storm like that you have three choices! 1) Find shelter 2) Find a quality umbrella not just the cheap one off the street or 3) Just get stormed on. Personally I have chosen 2, the quality umbrella, because this storm is here and there isn't any shelter. We have to go through it. Since umbrellas were not a thing of the old testament I chose the next best thing—God's wings.

> Have mercy on me, O God have mercy on Molly, for in you we take refuge, we will take refuge in the shadow of your wings until this storm has passed. Psalm 57:1

Next best thing to an umbrella, don't you think?

Today is Friday, if you would have told me that Molly would have gone out with her friends with things changing as they have, I would have fought you till the end... but there she went! Thank you, dear friends, for your prayers for her to have confidence. She grabbed up her courage put on her smile and went out with friends... maybe some of you don't think this is much but this is huge... our God is so big... and his mercies and grace are grander in this child than ever can be imagined! Maybe this is not the kind of update that you are expecting but this is life at God's best... it is the little steps that we take one in front of another and we just keep going... all of us!

If you are in a storm, what is your choice? I have got to say that being under God's wings is a pretty safe spot. He is the ultimate protector! How safe we are in God's arms—this is yet another tiny little light in our path and we are so very grateful! God is walking with us step by step and hearing your prayers...

With love,
Cathy

Praise God where ever you are and whatever situation He has allowed you to be in...His glory will shine through!

To: Cathy
From: Jo Ann
Sent: Friday, April 28

Dear Cathy,

What a PRAISE that Molly has "learned the secret of being content in any and every situation...and that she can do everything through him who gives her strength." Phil. 4:12, 13 going out with her friends today was a HUGE TESTIMONY to her confidence that can only come from the Lord! I am praying that she will continue to "be strong and take heart as she hopes in the Lord." Psalm 31:24 . . ."Let the beloved of the Lord—MOLLY—rest secure in Him, for He shields her all day long and the ONE the Lord loves—MOLLY—rests between His shoulders." Deut. 33:12 With much love and in much prayer for precious Molly and you and Mel and your whole family,

Jo Ann

To: Cathy
From: Barbi D
Sent: Friday, April 28

My prayer for Molly has been—"Give ear to my word, O Lord, consider my groaning. Hear the sound of my cry for help, my King and my God. For to thee do I pray. In the morning, O Lord, thou wilt hear my voice. In the morning I will order my prayers to thee and eagerly watch." Psalm 5:1–3

"For our light and momentary troubles are achieving for us an eternal glory that far out weighs them all." II Corinthians 4:17. Please tell Cathy and Molly that I am praying for their family daily.

Thanks,
Barbie

[A friend in bible study... I love the analogy of "momentary troubles"... if I could only grasp this as God does—momentary]

To: Cathy
From: Lindy
Sent: Friday, April 28

I know how much you hate facing those treatments, especially the strong ones. We will continue to be on our knees, Cathy, that she tolerates the drugs while they are killing off the bad cells. I pray she has an easy time and that the time will fly by and she will have it behind her in no time. Thanks for your updates and thanks to a God who does care.

Love,
Lindy

To: Cathy
From: Kay L
Sent: Saturday, April 29

Cathy, when you chose God's wings as your umbrella, you chose the best. He is the best umbrella! An umbrella made by man will only waste away. God Bless all of you and thanks for letting us know Molly is living her life in spite of this bump in the road. Shows so much about her character and where she puts her confidence... God alone. She is a witness to her friends and there is no telling the seeds she is planting. Everyone has bumps and she may be helping prepare someone that doesn't have the family she has to endure them.

Kay

To: Cathy
From: Linda B
Sent: Saturday, April 29

I do praise God. This is fabulous news. No one can tell us that God isn't still performing miracles! Kay L has been forwarding your emails and prayer requests, and this is just the news we wanted to hear. We'll keep praying. Tell Molly that several Houston gals are lifting her up daily, and we are thrilled with the answers. Love,

Linda B

[I have included this e-mail to show you an example of someone I don't know who is standing in the gap for Molly because she is a friend of a friend who cares. Many people were forwarding e-mails to people who were willing to pray. We didn't know then but were so grateful.]

To: Cathy
From: Kay S
Sent: Saturday, April 29

Cathy, it is almost as if God was sitting on the porch with us Thurs. and just listening to your deepest hurts and fears and then he arranged for Molly to have friends take her out Friday. Oh wait, that is EXACTLY what happened! I truly believe Friday was as much for her mom as her because I do believe your heart is breaking even more than she is suffering sometimes. That's what us moms do, isn't it, and then God comes in and takes over... can you imagine not having Him to FIX things for us? I am so thinking of you and

Mel and Molly, but more importantly, praying for each of the 3 of you. You are so walking his path and He is so going to plant flowers on your walk.

So Much Luv,
Kay

[Kay had come over on Thursday and we sat on the front porch. It was one of those days that she caught me at a low, a real low and sitting on the porch with a friend was the best medicine...I was glad she had come and appreciated her sweet heart as she listened to a hurting mom's heart]

To: Cathy
From: Gina
Sent: Saturday, April 29

Praise God for Molly's and Cathy's great attitude! "Knock and it shall be opened unto you." Matthew 7:7

> Thy hand be on the latch to open the door at His first knock. Shouldst thou open the door and not see Him, do not say He did not knock, but understand that He is there and wants thee to go out to Him. It may be He has something for thee to do for Him. Go and do it, and perhaps thou wilt return with a new prayer to find a new window in thy soul.—George MacDonald

Love,
Gina

To: Cathy
From: Beth
Sent: Saturday, April 29

How well we mother's know that our children's happiness makes us happy. I'm so thankful that Molly went out with her friends—- and blessings on those sweet friends for loving Molly! It is sometimes the small things that mean so much. God is faithful—-even in the small things.

Beth

[We became friends through our older daughters Brooke and Jamie, and have shared some fun times in Bunko and Bible study... she has always been an encourager]

To: Cathy
From: Allison
Sent: Saturday, April 29

Thanks for these amazing updates on Molly. I so thankful and blessed in knowing that we serve a Lord who is so concerned with our infirmities here on earth! I am praying for Molly that these next treatments will be not only powerfully effective but easily done, and that she will feel totally at peace throughout! "He who dwells in the shelter of the Most High will rest in the shadow of the Almighty" Ps.91:1

Love,
Allison

[This is a friend of Mary Leslie's who I have been blessed to hear from... she so has a love for the Lord and a gentle spirited gift of encouragement]

[Week six of treatments... May 1st... Halfway for the chemo part! We look back and think... we are trudging through this one step at a time. We are making our way to the end... and the best part is knowing there is an end! It is a slow process no doubt... and the effects of the chemo are mounting up causing fatigue... but Molly continues with her charm and determination and great tenacity.]

To: Kitty
From: Cathy
Sent: Monday, May 01
Subject: Molly Halfway through Chemo

We have made it halfway…6 down 6 to go…her blood counts were down today and if they don't pick up she will have to have an infusion next Monday. It won't be painful because everything is done through these PICC lines but it takes about 4 hours. Next week is a tough chemo week and we would appreciate your prayers for her body to somehow generate a healthy blood count report next Monday so she wouldn't have to be infused. We has an echogram and a pulmonary test this week on Wednesday to see how the chemo has affected her heart and her breathing.

Today we were at TCH and there was a little 6 year old boy crying and standing by the wall; his mom must have had to leave for a minute but I went and sat by him on the floor and asked him what was wrong? He said, "I want to stay." His counts were down and he was not able to have a treatment, yet he still wanted to stay! He had made friends, and this was a place that he could play with friends! Cancer was secondary.

Isn't it odd how we discern our priorities? So much is based on our experiences, our environment, our attitude and our needs. Where is my mindset? Colossians 3:2 Set your minds on things above not on earthly things, and Philippians 4:11 I need to be content in all circumstances. The mom came back a few minutes later; a young mom with a baby on her hip. My backpack just doesn't seem so heavy when I see the burdens so many others are carrying. But then I'm not Molly either… she is carrying a heavy load of her own… and she is doing it with such grace one day at a time!

As a side note: there is also another young 6 year old who has been at TCH at the same time we have been there on Monday's for treatments and he thinks he is Batman's right hand helper. He wears a black cape and flies around the infusion room making swishing sounds as he leaps from room to room. It is a terrific distraction and he really isn't noisy or imposing, just busy (he has cancer too)! But today I noticed something I hadn't seen in the past; he had words sewn on the bottom of his cape. He was flying too fast to read them so I asked his mom what they said. His grandmother has sewn on his cape the following words: Psalm 23:4, I will fear no evil, for God is with me...pretty much says it all... Don't you think? 6 year-old Batman mindset; No fear God is here!

Specific Prayer Request:
- Blood counts would be strong by next Monday
- Tests would show that heart and lungs are healthy
- We can scoot through the remaining 6 treatments without interruption and with good tolerance

Thank you for your prayers. It is with love and appreciation and a prayer back to God for blessings on your lives and on those you

Love.
Cathy

Praise God wherever you are and whatever situation He has allowed you to be in...His glory will shine through!

To: Cathy
From: Nancy
Sent: Monday, May 01

Cathy,
What a blessing to get this uplifting email from you. The Lord is certainly right there with you and Molly! What wonderful, faithful friends you have that keep praying to the Lord with such fervor and fortitude and faith. Molly and your family are ever in our prayers, as well

Love,
Nancy

[This is my cousin by marriage and what a blessing and encouragement she has been...but you have to read this knowing she has this wonderful southern draw when she speaks and a heart of gold]

To: Cathy
From: Kitty
Sent: Monday, May 01

"God that cannot lie promised" Titus 1:2. Faith is not working up by will power a sort of certainty that something is coming to pass, but it is seeing as an actual fact that God has said that this thing shall come to pass, and that it is true, and then rejoicing to know that it is true, and just resting because God has said it.

Faith turns the promise into a prophecy. While it is merely a promise it is contingent upon our cooperation. But when faith claims it, it becomes a prophecy, and we go forth feeling that it is something that must be done because God cannot lie. Taken from the devotional book, *Days of Heaven upon Earth* by A.B. Simpson:

> I hear men praying everywhere for more faith, but when I listen to them carefully, and get at the real heart of their prayer, very often it is not more faith at all that they are wanting, but a change from faith to sight. Faith says not, "I see that it is good for me, so God must have sent it," but, "God sent it, and so it must be good for me." Faith, walking in the dark with God, only prays Him to clasp its hand more closely.

Phillips Brooks:

> The Shepherd does not ask of thee
> Faith in thy faith, but only faith in Him;
> And this He meant in saying, "Come to me."
> In light or darkness seek to do His will,
> and leave the work of faith to Jesus

[I love the devotionals that Kitty would find and send]

To: Cathy
From: Jan G
Sent: Tuesday, May 02

My sweet friend and precious Molly—I prayed for you today as I read the following: When Shadrach, Meshach, and Abednego were thrown into the furnace, the fire did not stop them from moving, for they were seen "walking around." Actually, the fire was one of the streets they traveled to their destination. The comfort we have from Christ's revealed truth is not that it teaches us freedom from sorrow but that it teaches us freedom THROUGH sorrow!

I love you girls!
Jan G

To: Cathy
From: Susan H
Sent: Tuesday, May 02

Cathy...I ran across my ancient copy of Norman Vincent Peale's "Thought Conditioners."

Molly sought the Lord, and He heard her, and he delivered Molly from all her fears. Psalm 34:4

Thou wilt keep Molly in perfect peace, whose mind is stayed on Thee. Isaiah 26:3

Eye hath not seen, nor ear heard, neither have entered into the heart of man, the things which God hath planned for them that love Him. 1 Corinthians 2:9

Be strong, Molly, and of good courage: be not afraid, Molly; neither be thou dismayed: for the Lord thy God is with thee, Molly, whithersoever thou goest! Joshua 1:9

Please hold tight to the thought every night as you go to sleep that there are countless people praying for you and that through all these trials we all will witness God's mighty plan for your lives...He will be glorified...and he will use you for great things because you will be healed...so get ready!

[A bible study friend who had the wonderful ability of finding just the right verses and readings for encouragement]

To: Cathy
From: Kay L
Sent: Tuesday, May 02

Cathy, those were two great stories! Attitude and faith...so big! Cathy, continue to be used by God in this situation for sooooo many reasons. Molly is watching, others learn and receive comfort and encouragement, and most of all God is being glorified through your actions of kindness and compassion.

Love,
Kay

To:
From: Cathy
Sent: Sunday, May 07
Subject: The Last two day treatment

Well, tomorrow is our 7th out of 12 treatments. This is the last two day! We will go for chemo on Monday and Tuesday; Monday will be a tough day because her tests were cancelled for last Wednesday and two of them are rescheduled for this Monday.

Last week her counts were low and it was thought that she might have to have a blood transfusion as well on Monday but after talking to Dr. McClain, he said unless her counts drop unusually low this week then we will be able to continue this treatment and the regimen we are currently pursuing—(he is very conservative and the transfusions are only going to be given if her stamina is extremely low as well as the counts). He said that the chemo really starts effecting the body after this many treatments and we might possibly have to skip a week in lieu of a transfusion to help her body regroup on its own. My prayer is that we just keep on going and that her body somehow finds the strength to keep going the straight line without interruption for HER sake...

On a personal note: summer has hit and so many of her friends just want to go swimming She almost got thrown in the pool on Friday because you forget if you see her that anything is wrong because she looks just great—and they wanted her to swim. She has this PICC line in her arm (another thing disguised because she always wears these cute little jackets and the lines are always covered) and swimming is out... so as silly as this sounds please pray that she eases into summer with activities that are fun and is able to gently skirt the swimming issue without much attention or disappointment.

As far as thoughts that God has given me this week there are two of them—First of all, at church we have watched a film on two different occasions about our universe and galaxy and the sheer infinite spectrum of the realities of creation of God—then Mel and I went to the symphony on Friday night to hear music accompanying slides of the planets, that the symphony partnered with NASA to present, for a multi media presentation–

When God gives me a thought not once but twice especially in the same week I know he wants me to think about it a little harder—I have been thinking about it—and in my tiny little simple mind I often picture God sitting beside me in my car or in my living room and just talking with him as I would talk with you. I ask questions, vent concerns, cry a little, find some humor, praise him, but just most of all, I love it that I can be so comfortable interacting with Him, knowing that he is my friend. Then I see these cosmos pics, and I think, wait a minute. This seems to make God NOT so personal. So out of my simple shelf of reasoning—I think how can I bring into focus something simple that I could relate to from all of these overwhelming ideas and creations of God? Then it occurred to me, "THE STARS!" They are tangible! They are in the sight of my bounty of imaginings, and if God made the stars and God made me then we are somehow connected! Same creator... just way different scales! The stars are called to light up the sky; we are called to light up the world through Christ.

In Philippians 2:14–16—Do everything without complaining or arguing so that you may become blameless and pure children of

God without fault in a crooked and depraved generation, in which you shine like the stars of the universe—that I did not run or labor for nothing.

That's it—whatever you do, if you are doing it in the spectrum of obedience to God. Then you will shine like the stars, HIS stars! You will be one of them in this darkened world. The skies would not shine without stars nor would this world without the love of Christ shining through us. Am I shining or am I clouded by complaining? Whoops… So for now, I am going to try to keep all that is being done to care and to treat Molly in perspective. I am not going to complain but compliment what God has already done and what he has promised to do. I heard last week on Christian radio that instead of telling God about your problems, look at your problems and remind yourself who God is!

The second thought is anticipation. Why is that the anticipation of something either paralyzes us with worry or brightens our days with delight? What is it about anticipation that stirs our emotions and what is it that allows our behavior to be modified in one way or another? The answer lies in what it is that you believe about God! Is he REALLY a SOVEREIGN God? Or not?

> Ah, Sovereign LORD, you have made the heavens and the earth by your great power and outstretched arm. Nothing is too hard for you. Jeremiah 32:17

> But as for me, it is good to be near God. I have made the Sovereign LORD my refuge; I will tell of all your deeds. Psalm 73:28

> The Sovereign LORD is my strength; he makes my feet like the feet of a deer, he enables me to go on the heights. Habakkuk 3:19

So the next time I am dealing with anticipation or worrying about a test or a treatment, I am going to continue to try to remember that God is the Boss. He is the one making the calls. Only God! So why would I have anything in my heart but joy and expectation for what God will do next and... how he will reveal himself through circumstances that are certainly not in my control!

You don't have to read these you know or pass them on... these are just some thoughts of the week.

Thank you again for your continued prayers for Molly:

1) That she would be able to maintain sufficient blood counts and continue treatment without interruption
2) That the results of these two tests (lung and heart) would show that the drugs have not done any damage
3) That Molly's chemo treatments for Monday and Tuesday would continue to be tolerated and be effective
4) That Molly's attitude continues to be positive, her body strong
5) That we can move into summer without apprehension of activities

Please pray that Molly's counts are good enough for a treatment on Monday. We are 7 down, 5 to go. So close, and we are praying for safety for her body first and then hopefully no interruptions... of this regimen.

Cathy

Praise God wherever you are and whatever situation He has allowed you to be in... His glory will shine through!

[Week seven of treatment... May 8 I have been told that this protocol is producing very different responses than the ABVD protocol that is customarily used for Hodgkin patients at TCH. It seems to be easier on the body. The results are very encouraging and I think it will be truly considered for upcoming patients.]

To: Kitty
From: Cathy
Sent: May 8, 2006
Subject: Good Counts... What a Surprise

Kitty,

God continues to upset the expectations! Instead of Molly's counts being lower than last week they were higher. The only explanation is that the bone marrow is kicking in and raising the white blood cell count, and somehow her body is strong enough to rally! Dr. McClain did say that the drugs last week were NOT the heaviest hitters (it was an even week), and that too might have given her a little time to regroup. Whatever it was (and I think you and I know the real answer) it worked. God's healing hand of grace is upon this child—no doubt. When in the privacy of Dr. McClain and Mel and I and Molly was told she could let her guard down and say what she was really feeling; she stayed constant to her track and said "I am fine". He said, "Molly you do have a terrific attitude and you are just doing a fabulous job getting through this!" Again he is amazed.

I really would like to think that cooking a real dinner for four nights in a row including broccoli, spinach, and asparagus had its effect too... but that just isn't it! It did make Mel happy though.

It was a long day... but that is one more day done! She crashes each Monday about 4:00 p.m., her body just shuts down. The nausea thing is under control; what a blessing. The test results will be monitored within the week. We go in tomorrow for a short day. Thank you, dearly... but please remember to thank God for listening and being so obviously responsive. This is HIS doing you know... and HIS glory is shining through!

Cathy

Praise God where ever you are and whatever situation He has allowed you to be in... His glory will shine through!

To: Kitty
From: Cathy
Sent: Friday, May 12
Subject: Humility

This week was a tough week; Chemo Monday and Tuesday and the drugs resulted in what are often times called chemo-fatigue. I know I write this to so many of you who have been through these yourselves or have helped a dear friend and family member who has had to deal with this cancer issue. Until I had seen this side of the mountain I really had no idea or true understanding of the courage, the tenacity or perseverance that has resulted in the character of a patient or their family. I commend you... for you are the brave heroes of battle.

I write this note today regarding honor. I know Molly is really tired of this whole thing but she hardly ever says anything that is even near a complaint... she just keeps on trucking! This week she just felt awful and wanted to be quiet. She had no appetite, didn't want to visit and really just didn't want to be bothered... by anybody... me included. You know how you feel when your body is just yuck. I honored her request the best that I could, but I started thinking about what it is to be honored and why it is that we honor those that we do.

> Proverbs 15:33 The fear of the LORD teaches a man wisdom, and humility comes before honor.
>
> Proverbs 18:12 Before his downfall a man's heart is proud, but humility comes before honor.
>
> Proverbs 22:4 Humility and the fear of the LORD bring wealth and honor and life.
>
> Proverbs 29:23 A man's pride brings him low, but a man of lowly spirit gains honor.
>
> John 7:18 He who speaks on his own does so to gain honor for himself, but He who works for the honor

of the one who sent Him is a man of truth; there is nothing false about Him.

The reason we honor those that we do so often is because of their humility... and there it is in these verses in black and white. Molly has had a humble spirit throughout this whole ordeal. She has not been demanding or wimpy or self indulged. She has just quietly traveled down this road with perseverance, taking one day at a time and dealing with each obstacle in her own way with her own boundaries. It was a real flag for me to come to the realization of the times when I have wanted my own way and I have demanded honor.

No wonder I didn't get it. I was missing the humility part! I can't help thinking about the lessons that we are being taught in our family by watching not by hearing. She is only 16 but I know personally I have learned sometimes so much from what she hasn't said. I have watched as she has responded to each branch of this treatment in her own quiet spirit. This life hurdle jumped up and surprised all of us... But her humility has stood tall!

I am called to humble myself before the Lord and to humble myself before others. I just hate it when I get hit so hard over the head with my lifestyle. Pride, it just taps the worst in me and I ride it down the road. I have honored Molly and I honor God for the humility he showed through His Son. God so deserves to be honored every day and I have been so insufficient in doing that. What a lesson I am learning; by being the "mom" and not the "patient". I can't tell you how many times the frustration of self pride takes a front seat to humility. Change drivers! Change drivers! Change drivers! Maybe one day I will get this charge through my head and into my behavior.

Please pray that Molly's counts are good enough for a treatment on Monday. We are 7 down—5 to go—so close, and we are praying for safety for her body first and then hopefully no interruptions... of this regimen.

Thank you,
Cathy

Romans 12:10 Be devoted to one another in brotherly love. Honor one another above yourselves.

Ephesians 3:20 Now to him who is able to do immeasurably more than all we ask or imagine, according to his power that is at work within us.

Cathy

Praise God where ever you are and whatever situation He has allowed you to be in... His glory will shine through!

[Week eight of treatment–May 15]

To: Kitty
From: Cathy
Sent: Monday, May 15
Subject: Two months down... Yeah

We are down two months and one to go... Her counts were higher than they have been in several weeks and this was after tough chemo for two days; so we should be sailing through these next 4 weeks... we will skip a week when chemo is completed and then do radiation, which has been estimated for 2 weeks; each day, Mon. through Fri. May God's hand stay upon her... It is great to be on the downhill.

Thank you,
Cathy

Praise God wherever you are and whatever situation He has allowed you to be in... His glory will shine through!

To: Cathy
From: Gina
Sent: Monday, May 15

> Thou wilt keep her in perfect peace whose imagination is stayed on Thee. Isaiah 26:3

> Imagination is the greatest gift God has given us, and it ought to be devoted entirely to Him. —O. Chambers.

> Learn to associate ideas worthy of God with all that happens in Nature—the sunrises and the sunsets, the sun and the stars, the changing seasons, and your imagination will never be at the mercy of your impulses but will always be at the service of God." The Seeds of Thought Calendar—O. Chambers

[From Gina after being at the same symphony that Cathy mentioned last week]

To: Cathy
From: Kitty
Sent: Monday, May 15

Thank You, Lord that you arm Molly with strength and make her way perfect. 2 Samuel 22:33 Blessed is Molly whose strength is in You, Lord... She goes from strength to strength. Psalm 84:5, 7 Praise you, Lord, that Molly's hope is in the Lord and You will renew her strength. She will soar on wings like eagles She will run and not grow weary. She will walk and not be faint. Isaiah 40:31

Thank you, Lord, for your Word says: So do not fear, for I am with Molly. Do not be dismayed for I am her God. I will strengthen her and help her. I will uphold her with my right hand... For I am the Lord, your God, who takes hold Of her right hand and says to her, "Do not fear; I will help her.' Isaiah 41:10 & 13

Kitty

To: Cathy
From: Kitty
Sent: Friday, May 19

Attitude of Trust by Mrs. Charles E. Cowman
Taken from *Streams in the Desert:*

> "And it came to pass, before he had done speaking... and he said, Blessed be Jehovah... who hath not forsaken his loving kindness and his truth" (Gen. 24:15, 27). Every right prayer is answered before the prayer itself is finished—before we have "done speaking." This is because God has pledged His Word to us that whatsoever we ask in Christ's name (that is, in oneness with Christ and His will) and in faith, shall be done. As God's Word cannot fail, whenever we meet those simple conditions in prayer, the answer to our prayer has been granted and completed in Heaven as we pray, even though it's showing forth on earth may not occur until long afterward. So it is well to close every prayer with praise to God for the answer that He has already granted; He who never forsakes His loving-kindness and His truth. (See Daniel 9:20–27 and 10:12.)—Messages for the Morning Watch

> When we believe for a blessing, we must take the attitude of faith, and begin to act and pray as if we had the blessing. We must treat God as if He had given us our request. We must lean our weight over upon Him for the thing that we have claimed, and just take it for granted that He gives it, and is going to continue to give it. This is the attitude of trust. When the wife is married, she at once falls into a new attitude, and acts in accordance with the fact; and so when we take Christ as our Savior, as our Sanctifier, as our Healer, or as our Deliverer, He expects us to fall into the attitude of recognizing Him in the capacity that we have claimed, and expect Him to be to us all that we have trusted Him for.—Selected

The Final Round

Week nine of treatments... only three more after this one. Even though Molly is weary from the chemo, it gives us all a lift knowing that we can see the light at the end of HER tunnel. We have to keep focusing in that!

From: Cathy
Sent: Monday, May 22
Subject: Molly week 9

We are heading into our last month. Today will be a strong chemo day; I hesitated writing this note because I think everyone has got their own stuff and I thought you may be getting tired of hearing about ours... but several people this week have commented on how these e-mails have really been an encouragement to them so we will continue on. I know you will read them if you choose and delete them if they have gotten to be too much.

    I have thought often about this journey and the bumps and bruises we have gotten on the ride. I also have thought about the things we have seen that we might have missed if our fast pace of life had not been purposely slowed. This time with Molly has been a gift; as a sixteen year old you would never or most often not choose to be hanging out with your parents. Molly has held her own but she has also shown great respect and appreciation to us and for us.

    It makes me question how I relate to God. Do I respect him and appreciate him? Do I really trust him to make hard decisions for my life? Do I respect him when he says "no" or "wait"? Do I believe him when He says His ways are best? Do I really know he is standing beside me and will be there when I crater or am feeling alone and out of control?

Molly has had to depend on us. She has had to trust us. We had to depend on God and trust God. She hasn't had a choice but we have. It is with great thanksgiving that we knew God when things were going good so that when things got a little rocky, he was not a new friend; he was one who had already shown his colors!

Molly's life will be changed because of this. Her perspective on things and people and circumstances I suspect will be altered. How have I been changed? Subtly, but definitely. I hold all my children pretty close; as most of us do, but this was an "in my face" reminder that they are God's children first and are loaned to us. As much as I love Molly, God's love for her is abundantly more than I could ever imagine.

He uses each of us for his purposes–even our children—to help us grow into a deep relationship with him—a true friendship. This cancer that he has allowed Molly to have has unified a mighty force of prayer warriors for the purpose of praying for perfect healing. It has impacted my family, each one of us, and we are watching as God's mighty hand is revealed through answers to prayers. Your prayers and our prayers are being heard but more importantly our relationship with GOD IS GROWING. I know mine is growing and yours is too- IT MIGHT BE SUBTLE BUT we all ARE CHANGING!

God is working–In the movie The Chronicles of Narnia, there is only one thing that the white witch is afraid of and doesn't want to hear... and it is this: "Asylan is on the move!" God is on the move! A situation like this makes you keenly aware that you need someone strong and mighty and wise in your arena; someone who loves you in an uncompromising way, someone who you know will always have your best interest in mind, and someone who is not scared to let you go through something hard to make you someone better.

This IS hard and hopefully God is teaching me to be better because of it. One thing I have learned is "know where to focus" and "know who to focus on". Each time I have changed the focus to me, each time... it has resulted in fear or disappointment or judgment of others, or unrest... each time! I know that is a lesson for me that has been highlighted (like one of those yellow highlighters that make a certain point stand out) and God is good to make that lesson clear. It won't change today or tomorrow but it will improve… and it will be subtle.

Molly has weathered this storm in a great way but I think she is probably about ready for this whole deal to be through. Though we only have 4 treatments left including this one, please pray that she would continue to hang in there. She wants to be invisible and is not too good with attention. I think that she really cannot fathom the number of people she is affecting… those who are praying as well as those who God is blessing because of their prayers. Psalm 31: 7 you are my hiding place, you will protect me from trouble—she wants to just blend in—and not be the different one—she has been exempted from all finals except history—and she will take that on Thursday at home- the last day of school—then summer. And summer will have its own challenges—because we will be dealing with this till mid July.

Please pray that these last weeks will go fast and that there will be some fun around the corner and we will be able to find joy in each day and praise in each circumstance.

I praise God that when we have called He has answered. Psalm 138:3, 8: When I called you answered me; you made me bold and stouthearted. The Lord will fulfill his purpose for me.
Thank you dear friends! Expect to see God's hand today on your life and on those you love,

Cathy

> Isaiah 49:13 For the Lord comforts his people and will have compassion on his afflicted ones.
>
> May you arm Molly with strength to complete this journey—Psalm 18:30 You armed me with strength for battle.
>
> Thank you again for your continued prayers.

Praise God wherever you are and whatever situation He has allowed you to be in... His glory will shine through!
To: Cathy
From: Lindy
Sent: Monday, May 22
Subject: Molly week 9

I just read your last email about people being tired of hearing about you. I cannot tell you how much your emails have meant to me. I hope I am not overstepping my bounds by writing to you directly but I just felt compelled to do so. You really are pursuing this task, arm in arm with God and that is just how we are supposed to live every moment of every day. Molly will do something so wonderful with this. I can only imagine the lives she will touch along her path. (She already has). And you, Cathy, are imparting amazing glimpses of God's grace, even in the darkest of times, you are remaining faithful and I know you will be blessed by this.

I thank you for sharing yourself, you heart, your Molly, your life with us. You are making a difference... a big one!

Love,
Lindy

[What a sweet and dear friend... and what an encouragement]

To: Cathy
From: Terri S
Sent: Monday, May 22

Cathy, God loves your dialog with your friends who love you and your family. We are learning and growing along with you. When we pray we pray that His power is shown in our situation. God is so happy to hear our group prayers and see us joined in His praise and glory. Thank you for sharing with us. It is a ministry in itself.

Love,
Terri

[This is another friend from a past bible study... she faithfully would send me notes and each one of them meant so much]

To: Cathy
From: David S
Sent: Monday, May 22

Cathy, Your email was forwarded to us. I read every word and would be honored if you put us directly on your email list so that we can know specifically what to pray for. Please know that true loving and caring brothers and sisters in Christ will not tire of your emails. Those of us who have gone through trauma and trials like this have empathy. We feel your pain. We truly and genuinely care and love you and desire to come along side you (for Molly's sake, quietly), to lift you up and to pray for Molly and your family. Your family is precious to us and the church.

Cathy, you blessed me a couple of years ago at a KA function recalling then how tough you felt my losses must have been. They were very tough and those times I really wondered if God really did not give us challenges that were greater than we could endure. Oh, how I was stretched and so sad and how I said in anger to God "How dare the Bible say; "Rejoice in your suffering"? But do you know what? It was in the curiosity of exploring just what that verse meant that got me on the other side of my trials and grief. It was the simple but difficult application of understanding that our suffering is a progressive process which leads us to finding our true significance and "Hope" in HIM. A hope that is not "temporal," but a hope that is eternal and does not disappoint us.

Oh, the persevering and character building part of that progression is so tough and unbearable it seems at times. You will persevere, you will be made stronger, and you will get through it... My prayer for you folks is that you can rest in the fact that God is sovereign. He guides our steps daily. He is a healing God. May you be comforted by our prayers. May the Lord bless you folks and keep you strong and steady. May He daily make His face shine upon you and give you a peace that passes all our understanding. May He give you rest.

God bless you,
David.

[This is a long time friend from church. Our families have worshipped together since our children were born. We have walked the same path on many occasions. These thoughts were such a blessing to me. It was such a reminder to me that we all need to hold each other up because everybody has something!]

To: Kitty
From: Cathy
Sent: Tuesday, May 23
Subject: The Battle is Raging

There is this measure by which the doctors and nurses go by called an ANC! Each week it is measured by a bunch of different itemized things blended together then averaged out and that is how they decide if Molly's body is up for the treatment. Last week I said her counts were higher than they had been in weeks. The ANC was, and I thought (shows you I still know so little) that this was the beginning of wonderful news and for this week and the next treatments and the counts would not even be an issue. WRONG! Her counts especially white blood counts have dropped dramatically... still able to have treatment but on the really low side. No explanation except the drugs are powerful and the battle is still raging though the tests have shown the cancer to be tackled.

Dr. McClain said he has never had a patient go through the entire protocol without taking a pause for a week or so (the protocol he is speaking of is the TCH one and not the Stanford V that we are on... they didn't know what to expect on Stanford V) and to not be concerned if we need to take a break. When he told me that, at the beginning of these treatments, my prayer was, "God, you can take us through this without interruption. If it is your will, please let us ride the straight line. Three treatments left and I still am asking God to not interrupt this and keep Molly safe and her body strong. "Let's just get this behind us...

for the sake of this precious child." Only one of the remaining treatments is a really heavy one. The other two are very tolerable. Psalm 112:7 He (a righteous man) will have no fear of bad news; his heart is steadfast trusting in the Lord.

She is sick today and weak! We had a PET exam this am at 7:00 and she had to leave her stomach empty too long. Gosh, I can't stand to be so helpless and stand by and watch as she hurts and just plain feels crumby. Still no complaints from her, you can just see how she feels by the look on her face. I keep thinking…this too will pass! But please let it pass quickly. Probably by evening. Every day is one more day down…I admire the perseverance of those of you who are having to wrestle with: establishing what is wrong, or looking for a diagnosis or dealing with a long term illness. That must be so very hard. One of my praises is that this disease has been identified and researched and is curable. I am greatly thankful if she has to have cancer that it was this particular one; for as horrible of an ordeal as it is, we can confidently see a successful end and then a new beginning.

There are two things that occurred to me the past few days! The first was when I was in my closet dressing…this was merely a pondering thought rather than a practical life application.

Yesterday I thought, *Here we are on Monday morning, same weekly schedule as many Mondays before. Here I am getting dressed to take my 16 year old daughter to chemo. She has cancer; the reality of it seems so surreal. Then I thought of everybody else getting dressed for their day. Some are going to work, some are getting to spend a day with their parents, some are exercising, some are playing golf, some are having lunch with a friend, some are going to hospitals, some are on vacation and the world is out there moving.*

Though our activities differ, we all are able to clothe ourselves with similar characteristics:

> I Colossians 3:12 Therefore, as God's chosen people, holy and dearly loved, clothe yourselves with compassion, kindness, humility, gentleness and patience.
>
> Isaiah 51:9—clothe yourself with strength.

Whatever the day holds we are all told to be wearing the same things. Our reasons for getting dressed will be different but our attitudes are called to be similar. If I could just remember to clothe myself as I have been taught!

The second thought as I was taking Molly for her PET exam was:

My dad and his wife, Wilhelmina, are quite the movers (and they are in their 80's). They just like to be on the go and each of us has the opportunity to go to different events with them. When we go to the football game or the baseball game, or any event for that matter, there are usually at least two of us and we flank them as they walk in so that the crowds are kept from bumping into them. Of course, we do this very subtly, but in our own way we try to protect them from unintentional bombardment.

I was thinking about Molly today and how Mel and I have tried to flank her. Then it came to me: I believe in the TRINITY of God; the Father, the Son and the Holy Spirit. A dramatic vision came before me of being flanked by the Father and the Son and being led by the Holy Spirit. For a moment that thought made me seem invincible. How could you lose? Or be bombarded? For there was protection on all sides and these protectors were not your ordinary bodyguards. They were divine spirit guards. Then, as Peter lost his focus when he was walking on water, so did I. This protection scenario is something that I think merits remembrance in my heart on a moment by moment basis.

I am flanked! What a gift that God has promised. Not just some obscure gesture of presence, but a reality of God in his person and spirit, just as God was with Isaac.

> Gen 26:24 Don't be afraid, I am with you, and was with Joshua.
>
> Joshua 3:7 I am with you as I was with Moses.
>
> John 16:32 I am not alone—my Father is with me.

I am not alone! Neither are any of us! Lonely sometimes, but not alone. Flanked we are! We should think about that the next time we see danger or fear coming our way. I would just love that if I could make that a habit! Wouldn't you?

Cathy
Praise God where ever you are and whatever situation He has allowed you to be in...His glory will shine through!

To: Cathy
From: Tommy G
Sent: Tuesday, May 23

This is my favorite "being flanked" set of verses. Psalm 121:

> 1 I lift up my eyes to the hills—
> From whence comes my help?
> 2 My help comes from Yahweh,
> the maker of heaven and earth.
> 3 May He not allow your foot to be moved;
> May He who protects you not slumber.
> 4 Behold, He who keeps Israel
> shall neither slumber nor sleep.
> 5 Yahweh is your keeper;
> Yahweh is your shade over your right hand.
> 6 The sun shall not strike you by day,
> nor the moon by night.
> 7 Yahweh will keep you from all calamity;
> He will keep your soul.
> 8 Yahweh will protect your going out and your coming
> in, from this time forth, and even forevermore.

[This was Molly's soccer coach in middle school and is one of my friend's who shares a love for Oswald Chambers...we have been blessed to have he and his wife Julie involved with our youth group at our church, CEPC.]

To: Cathy

From: Jill
Sent: Tuesday, May 23

Precious Cathy, your e-mails to us are Holy Spirit inspired. "As thy days, so shall thy strength be. The eternal God is thy refuge, and underneath are His everlasting arms, and He shall thrust out the enemy from before thee…" Deuteronomy 33:25b, 27 Molly is ever before us in prayer.

I love you,
Jill

[anyone who calls me precious… what a heart]

To: Kitty
From: Cathy
Sent: Thursday, May 25
Subject: Cheer

I bought a new picture for the back of my stairs as a reminder to all of us who travel those stairs: It says: "The Best of all Healers is good Cheer". A few days later on my walk the words "Be of Good Cheer" were a constant chant on my mind. I had asked the Lord to walk with me and guide my thoughts. What a simple thought he gave me, and kept giving me. Cheer is the best healer. Think of the last time someone said something cheerful to you, or even just represented cheer with a smile. It does do something to your countenance: it lifts you. No matter how low or sad or anxious, it somehow brings a little boost to your day.

I think of how many times many of you have sent good cheer to us; thoughtful phone calls, e-mails, little note, etc., and it is the BEST HEALER. For Good Cheer is a product of Joy. Don't you think? And a cheerful look does bring JOY to the heart. May you be of good cheer this Memorial Day Weekend. And may God keep you safely in the palm of his hands.

Proverbs 12:25 An anxious heart weighs a man down, but a kind word cheers him up.

Proverbs 15:13 A happy heart makes the face cheerful, but heartache crushes the spirit.
Proverbs 15:30 A cheerful look brings joy to the heart, and good news gives health to the bones.

Proverbs 17:22 A cheerful heart is good medicine, but a crushed spirit dries up the bones.

Love,
Cathy

Praise God wherever you are and whatever situation he has allowed you to be in...His glory will shine through.

To: Cathy
From: Jan G
Sent: Thursday, May 25

My sweet friend...I love you so very much—you are continuously in my heart and in my prayers. I read your "e's" over and over and find them a tremendous source of encouragement and inspiration. I am in awe of your strength and amazing ability to express your heart through the written word. I am quite sure you have no idea the powerful effect you have on each of us. God breathes His Word through you and you so elegantly share it with all of us. You are a walking demonstration to this world that Satan is a defeated foe! I thought of you as I read this "He has thrown open to you His exhaustive treasury. Go in and draw upon Him in simple childlike faith, and you will never again have the need to rely on anything else." This is you! God's grace and glory is being revealed in your life and you are letting your light shine to all who know you! Jacob won the victory and the blessing not by wrestling with his circumstances, but by clinging to God (Gen. 32: 26, 29). Molly is covered in prayer from the top of her beautiful head to the soles of her feet!

Jdg

[Just so you will know these big thoughts come from a tiny framed little angel who has the grandest smile]
To: Kitty
From: Cathy
Sent: Friday, May 26
Subject: Stay Beside Me Bentley

Molly's new dog Bentley is learning to take walks in the neighborhood. Mel and I walk 2 or 3 nights a week and have started taking both dogs with us... We also have a sweet 12 year old lab named Khaki. This week Mel said try to keep Bentley on your right. We turned off Memorial and took her off the leash and she followed pretty well. We have a route that we take but because Bentley is still little we can't go the whole route. I said, "Lets at least follow this first phase of our walk so she'll know the routine." Mel said it isn't important that she knows the routine but that it is more important that she knows to stay with you and follow you. I have been walking the dogs each morning and he's right. I have changed the routine, the path... but Bentley is learning to stay beside me (with only a little bit of wandering) without a leash. And Khaki, our older dog learned this a long time ago, so she never has a leash, even on Memorial.

I think you pretty much know where I'm going with this. On my walk this morning, as Bentley followed close, I thought God doesn't want me to get used to the same routine, He just asks that I follow Him, wherever He leads.

I get up with Bentley, feed him, wash his mat, and play with him. He trusts me. God gets up with me, supplies my needs, and is my constant companion and I trust him. So when there is no leash (accountability) making me stay on path, I too have that choice. Do I follow and stay close or wander? Oh, I wander. But just like Bentley, I always have my Master in sight and come running a little faster now when I'm called. John 10:27 "My sheep listen to my voice. I know them and they follow me."

Molly has finished finals, school is over. Yeah! She is feeling great for the weekend. Thank you, dear friends, so very much for your continued prayers.

Cathy

Praise God wherever you are and whatever situation He has allowed you to be in... His glory will shine through!

[Week 10 of treatments... still praying for a straight line]

To: Kitty
From: Cathy
Sent: Tuesday, May 30
Subject: Molly Has Low Blood Counts

Today is the first time Molly has requested that I ask my friends to pray for her. I have asked her if she wanted to read e-mails, responses, etc. and her answer has always been "No." She is sooooo PRIVATE and the idea that this story about HER is so out there is for the world to see is a little disconcerting. But today she finally made me realize that she does trust your prayers to be effective and though she has always appreciated them, she just doesn't want to talk about this whole deal or have anyone else talk about it either. Hard to be on the fence, need the help, trust the helpers and want to be silent too. Something has to give... and she finally did!

Her counts were the lowest ever today, and if it had been an odd week we would not have gotten treatment. This drop has to be monitored so we have to go back on Friday specifically to have blood counts reevaluated. If she has continued to drop she will possibly need a blood transfusion.

This is the deal: most often after an even week her body gets a little time to regroup (we are in an even week so there is hope that her body will compensate on its own) but towards the end of a chemo protocol (we are down to the last 2 treatments) the drugs have taken a beating on the body and it is just tired. The transfusion will take about 4 hours and it will be done at TCH. I donated blood today and it will be available for 30 days but the thing is...

she doesn't want to sit there for 4 hours (it won't hurt; they will use her PICC line). It just isn't something she wants to sit and do. (Imagine that)

This is when she said, "MOM, WILL YOU ASK YOUR FRIENDS TO PRAY FOR THIS PLEASE!" I know I gave her the biggest smile of appreciation... for she keeps things so tucked away and she finally acknowledged that she has trusted these prayers and has depended on them. So I am asking you to please pray for the specific prayers listed below.

We have been walking through this journey for such a short time compared to so many battles that others face. Even through these short battles in comparison to others, you get a little anxious and wonder if you can hold on and stay positive and keep your attitude in check for the duration. You get restless and your spirits are worn thin.

I have been reading a book by David Jeremiah called a Bend in the Road (a book recommended to me by Lynda T. at the beginning of this cancer journey). He has written a wonderful chapter on Psalm 13 talking about when God delays. It is about David asking God how much longer this will go on. At the end of the Psalm he is singing a song of Thanksgiving. I will sing to the Lord because he has dealt bountifully with me. We are singing to the Lord and praising him for his mighty works.

But, as I write this I am thinking about the T's. They must be asking the same questions of God that David did. "How much longer?" Rebekah's (age 19) cancer has come back for yet another time. Please ask God to comfort this precious family and help them see this as David did. When anxiety for the future built up, and it did time and again, David faced it with the testimony of the past. God has attacked this cancer before with success. Let him attack it again once and for all and let his mighty hand rest upon Rebekah and her family. GOD is listening to his people as they pray for her healing. May His will be done and may His purpose be declared as He unfolds His grace through this trial.

The T's are dear friends and have been such a comfort and encouragement to all of us from the moment we shared our news of Molly. I know God allows us the fiery trials so we can be there to help others when they experience a similar battle. They have been there. Who would have thought that we would be asking for God's mighty hand of healing again for them? But we are... and He is listening I know.

Specifically for Molly:
1) Please pray that her counts go up and rise to the level of acceptance for her last tough treatment (she has two treatments left but the one next week is a two day, Mon. and Tues. and it is the most intense—another treatment will follow on the next Monday and that will be her last chemo)
2) Please pray that we continue to be on an uninterrupted protocol.
3) Keep her safe from viruses and bacteria as her immune system is very weak
4) She has a CT scan this week (this was the one she had such a hard time with last month). Please pray that she will be able to deal with that yucky stuff that she has to swallow (there is so much of it).
5) Pray that the PET scan results showed that the cancer has been tackled in full; no trace.
6) AND PLEASE pray for Rebekah and her family as they courageously go into battle once again. Pray for tenacity, courage, comfort, peace and rest from anxious hearts and thoughts and please Lord, shield them from discouragement and fear.

Thank you so much, with love and appreciation not just from me, from Molly too! We are ever so grateful!

Cathy

Praise God wherever you are and whatever situation He has allowed you to be in...His glory will shine through!

To: Cathy
From: Kitty
Sent: Tuesday, May 30

Cathy, as usual you touched my heart with your message you sent out today. Please see below a sweet message from Nita. I look forward to seeing you tomorrow and praying together. I think we should sing a song of thanksgiving as God inhabits our praises. May Jehovah Rapha, The Great Healer, do a mighty work in Molly this week.

Love,
Kitty

To: Cathy
From: Lisa
Sent: Tuesday, May 30

Cathy,

I am so glad I receive the emails about Molly. I continue to pray for her daily and think of her sweet spirit a lot! She came to our house last night to be with her friends and I think she had a good time. Molly is so gorgeous, and sweet! What a sweet daughter you have! I just hugged her and want her to be healed! I know she will be! She does shine, Cathy! What a blessing of a child you have! I just look at her and she shows happiness even after all that she has been through (and I don't even know how much!). I don't know if I could even be that good. It sure makes me look at my own life a lot harder and be more thankful for everything I have.

I loved seeing her last night and I am glad she came over! If there is anything I can do, Please let me know! GOD will heal her! I just know it!

Many, Many Prayers! AND LOVE,
Lisa Cunningham

[This a friend who has a daughter in Molly's class...we carpooled before the girls were driving and now only see each other once in a while...I loved hearing about Molly from someone else who had seen her]

[The following e-mail is a forward from Gina about Rebekah T. Lynda and I each are on familiar ground with our daughters having cancer and being about the same ages. As moms, our hearts are torn as we watch and are unable to take away the torment of this disease. The battle that Lynda is watching Rebekah fight has raged a greater war and they have had to address an uncertain path of treatment. We pray for each other often... and there is empathy and compassion deep within each of our hearts that words cannot express... It is felt through an unseen bond with Christ.]

To: Cathy
From: Gina and Lynda
Sent: Tuesday, May 30
Subject: Rebekah's report

Dear Gina,

I cannot even come close to expressing the lifelong blessing you have given to me by organizing a group of friends to pray for my daughter and our family through this. My cup overflows. I want to be able to attend Bible Study but cannot tomorrow. I wanted you to have the first ups on what is going on.

First and foremost, thankfulness, worship, and praise for how good God is.

Today we spent from 10–2 at the hospital and got nothing accomplished. This is very unusual as they needed to wait for blood results before they started tests. Since Mon. was a holiday, after 3 hours they still did not have her results. We left.

Tomorrow we go from 8-after 2. She has chest, head, and neck pet scans, other scans, and meeting with surgeon at 2. Our 1st doctor retired and now we have a younger one. Not as experienced but with the team of doctors he should work well. Our Dr. Raney, called today and said if it hasn't spread anywhere else this was good. Most times when it reappears it does so all over. Thank Jesus we have not had that and are praying it is localized in her neck in just the small tumor. With this new treatment they may not remove it but use it as a gage to see how effective the chemo works. She will be taking 1 hour of chemo 5 days a week for 2 weeks and then off a week. So 2 out of 3 weeks she will go to hospital for 1–2 hours, 5 days a week. They say the only side effect is diarrhea which sounds promising. The dr. said if she was bent on going to school they could get in 3 treatments. We just haven't discussed much since we don't have the tests yet. Please, Lord Jesus, may this be localized and easy to eliminate.

Will let you know more after tomorrow. Today was a great day afterwards. We went and had lunch and shopped a little. A friend of hers went with us.

I love you Gina and thank you,
Lynda

To: Cathy
From: Lynda
Sent: Thursday, June 1

Cathy, You are the most precious person I have ever met. You are as cute as can be. I feel sorry for people that don't know you and am sooooooooo thankful I dooooooooo!

Stayed home today and slept. Last 2 days at hospital are draining but we manage to have fun. Leaving tomorrow for Ft. Worth. Rebekah wants to go to orientation for TCU. May get 3 treatments in and then go to school. Not sure what is going on. I am praying for Jesus to zap it out. Have you read John 9 lately? It will make you feel good.

Any change with Molly? I hope to get to know her someday soon.

Want to see you and be with you. Wish we could go with you tomorrow night but leaving for Ft. Worth in afternoon. Will be back Tues. Don't know what next week holds but hope to see you and come to Gina's on Wed.

Love you!
Lynda

[I hesitated including this first part but it so shows you her personality and her encouragement and why I love her so much]

To: Cathy
From: Lynda
Sent: Thursday, June 1

Hi. It's me again. I just read your e-mail about Molly's transfusions. We too are praying that her blood levels will come back up. Is it for blood or platelets? We had numerous ones of both. It came to be pretty routine. She will feel much better afterwards if she has one. They also give you something that makes you sleepy. You also don't need to worry about bad blood. The screening criteria in the last few years rules out anything scary.

Love again,
Lynda

To: Kitty
From: Cathy
Sent: Friday, June 2
Subject: Molly's Upcoming Tests

Kitty,
    Mel is out of town and I just woke up with a bunch of anxious thoughts this morning. We have a CT scan this morning and a Pulmonary (lung) later in the day and then blood counts. Part of it is knowing how anxious Molly is and wanting to smooth that over. And part of it is teetering on the fence wondering what God's will really is...
    So I put my walking shoes on and gathered the dogs and decided to ask him. In a short while these were the words... I CAN AND I WILL! I'm not really sure what God was responding to for there have been so many requests; only that he can and he will today...

He'll get her through this day. He will handle the counts and then it will be done! It gets down to; do I believe that God is able to do this? And do I have faith that he will? I am answering "Yes!" And look forward to the events of the day! It is pretty fine knowing I can just send this out and she will be lifted in prayer—once again my thanks.

Love,
Cathy

> 2 Corinthians 9:8 and God is able to make all grace abound to you, so that in all things at all times, having all that you need, you will abound in every good work.
>
> Philippians 3:21 who, by the power that enables him to bring everything under his control, will transform our lowly bodies so that they will be like his glorious body
>
> Matthew 9:27-29
> 27As Jesus went on from there, two blind men followed him, calling out, "Have mercy on us, Son of David!" 28When he had gone indoors, the blind men came to him, and he asked them, "DO YOU BELIEVE THAT I AM ABLE TO DO THIS?" "Yes, Lord," they replied. 29Then he touched their eyes and said, "According to your faith will it be done to you";

Praise God wherever you are and whatever situation He has allowed you to be in...His glory will shine through!

To: Cathy
From: Kitty
Sent: Friday, June 2
Subject: Bible Verses

Yesterday a group met a Gina home to pray for Molly and Rebekah. Everyone shared verses and these were the ones we read. Philippians 1:2–6... For I am confident of this very thing, that He who began a good work in Molly and Rebekah will perfect it until the day of Christ Jesus Romans 12:12 Rejoicing in hope, persevering in tribulation, devoted to pray.

Psalm 119:17–19, 26–27 (From the Living Bible) Bless Molly and Rebekah with life so that they can continue to obey you. Open their eyes to see wonderful things in your Word. They are but pilgrims here on earth: how they need a map, and your commands are their chart and guide. I told you their plans and you replied. Now give them instructions. Make them understand what you want, for then they shall see your miracles

Isaiah 43:1–2 Do not fear, for I have redeemed Molly and Rebekah; I have called them by Name; they are 'Mine! When they pass through the waters, I will be with them; And through the rivers, they will not overflow them. When they walk through the fire, they will not be scorched. Nor will the flame burn them. For I am the Lord their God.

Jeremiah 29:11–14 For I know the plans that You have for Rebekah and Molly, declares the Lord, plans to prosper them and not to harm them, to give them a future and a hope. Then they will call upon me and come and pray to me, and I will listen to them. And they will seek me and find me, when they search for me with all their heart...

Philippians 4:4–7 Rejoice in the Lord always; again I will say, rejoice!... Be anxious for nothing, but in everything by prayer and supplication with thanksgiving let your requests be made know to God. And the peace of God, which surpasses all understanding, shall guard their hearts and their minds in Christ Jesus.

Kitty

[I love it when specific names are inserted in scriptures]

To: Cathy
From: Jan G.
Sent: Friday June 2
Subject: I can and I will

Good morning by sweet friend! "I Can and I Will!" Well, that about says it all! I love the fact that you put on your walking shoes and gathering your little buddies and just headed out, knowing that He is just waiting to talk to you, to reveal Himself in ways that are completely unique to you. What glory! Being a King's Kid has definite advantages! Cathy, I love you so much and carry you in my heart constantly. You are brave and strong; you truly are a warrior in every sense of the word. Through your heart thoughts, you are leading all of us in this battle. Your unwavering faith in our Abba Father encourages and inspires each of us to continue to put our trust in the One who says, "I CAN and I WILL!" Molly is in the shelter of the Most High; she is in His palm; she is covered from the top of her head to the soles of her feet as we plead the blood of Jesus over her. "I CAN and I WILL..."AMEN!

Love,
Jan

To: Cathy
From: Suzanne M
Sent: Saturday, June 3
Subject: Prayer

Cathy, just to let you know... I am praying for Molly... all throughout the day. Thanks for these updates. They really give me specifics for prayer for her. June 2 devotion in Streams in the Desert is wonderful. Romans 4: 18–19 Against all hope, Abraham in hope believed... Without weakening in his faith... the writing goes on to explain how great strong faith is only accomplished through enduring great trials. Thank you for your sharing with all of us how God is sustaining you and your family through your great trial... Let me know whenever you will be ready to grab a cup of coffee... Love to Molly...

Love you,
Suzanne

To: Cathy
From: Kitty
Sent: Saturday, June 3
Subject: Devotional

Streams in the Desert
Author: Mrs. Charles E. Cowman
Program Date: June 3rd, 2000

"Let us pass over unto the other side" (Mark 4:35).

Even when we go forth at Christ's command, we need not expect to escape storms; for these disciples were going forth at Christ's command, yet they encountered the fiercest storm and were in great danger of being overwhelmed, so that they cried out in their distress for Christ's assistance.

Though Christ may delay His coming in our time of distress, it is only that our faith may be tried and strengthened, and that our prayers may be more intense, and that our desires for deliverance may be increased, so that when the deliverance does come we will appreciate it more fully.

Christ gave them a gentle rebuke, saying, "Where is your faith? Why did you not shout victory in the very face of the storm, and say to the raging winds and rolling waves, 'You can do no harm, for Christ, the mighty Savior is on board?'"

It is much easier to trust when the sun is shining than when the storm is raging.

We never know how much real faith we have until it is put to the test in some fierce storm; and that is the reason why the Savior is on board.

Sweet Sixteen with Hodgkins 119

If you are ever to be strong in the Lord and the power of His might, your strength will be born in some storm.

"With Christ in the vessel, I smile at the storm." Christ said, "Let us go to the other side"—not to the middle of the lake to be drowned.—Dan Crawford

To: Cathy
From: Kristy
Sent: Sunday, June 4

Hi, my little friend. I have just gotten home this evening and have been so anxious to see how Friday went. I am glad to have specific things to pray for and know that God is and will be right in the middle of everything... even a parking place for school next year! Wow! I will be praying hard that Molly stays well, has increased white cells, and finds strength and joy from just hanging out at home. I'll also be praying for God's strength, comfort and peace for you and all your family. Love you all!

Kristy

[This is my dear friend for all seasons... and I too am her friend for all seasons. She was the one who God used to encourage and nudge me to mail this document to a publisher. We meet at least once a month for a hamburger, French fries and a coke and work through some of life's challenges at hand... we cry a little and laugh a lot and then rejoice for the time God carved out for us to meet. She is a blessing in my life... and by the way SHE is the little one, truly little... and her opening of "Hi, my little friend" is my most affectionate greeting... and it is always her greeting to me, not just a here or there comment.]

[Summary: Week 11 of treatments... June 5... we are almost through with the chemo; this is when you wish that that would be the end... especially since the tests have shown so good and positive... I have tried to dodge the radiation issue with Dr. McClain but he said that one of the primary reasons that this protocol has been so effective is that you have to "treat" according to the rules... if you forgo the rules then there the percentages change... for the percentage of 90% cured is based on the whole treatment and we have to stick to it...]

To: Kitty
From: Cathy
Sent: Monday, June 5
Subject: Molly's 11th Treatment

Today we had an excellent appointment with Dr. McClain. Though her counts were still down; her white counts had doubled since Friday—Molly was not able to get chemo because white cells are still too low but they were high enough to ward off an immunity injection and the red cells were high enough to dodge a transfusion—Dr. McClain is encouraged to think that a couple of days will give her the required blood levels so Wednesday and Thursday will her designated days this week.

This morning in Oswald Chambers he quoted Hebrews 13:5 –6—I will not leave you or forsake you and the Lord is my helper I will not fear... There is just something in our natural emotional gut that allows that fear to seep in through the cracks - and it takes a constant mental presence to ask God to ward it off..

I received this e-mail from Jan G. when I got home this afternoon and she nailed it...

> Do not despair! When you are weak from the fierce fires of severe trials do not be tempted to despair. Do not try to be strong. Just "be still and know that He is God." Be still and KNOW that He WILL sustain you and bring you through the fire. "I would have despaired unless I had believed that I would see the goodness of the Lord... Wait for the Lord; be strong, and let your heart take courage." Psalm 27:13–14 "We went through fire and water, but you brought us to a place of abundance." Psalm 66:12
>
> You're in my heart,
> Jan

Sometimes you just have to BE STILL AND KNOW...God is faithful and Big and in charge of this whole picture...He will bring us through the fire—but he will do it his way...so far he has done it in a way that has been a revelation to Dr. McClain—he said today that he has never had a patient be this strong and weather this disease as Molly has...he can not believe the way she looks or feels and is truly amazed...Your prayers have been honored—and God has given Molly the grace and strength and tenacity to fight this battle—I know that there are many of you reading this e-mail that are fighting your own battles—it might be health related, relational, financial, job related or just plain life itself—but whatever it is—please know first that you are not alone...just ask God to come along beside you—and carry that heavy backpack—you will be amazed at the folks he will put in your path to remind you of his presence—the things that they will say and do will knock your socks off—and second take time to:

BE STILL—in this crazy world that we live in we are constantly on the go and trying to wade through distractions and solve issues be big or small—just remember to take time to be quiet—and find something good and excellent (Philippians 4:8 & 9) to fill your mind and replace anxious thoughts of fear or indecision or discomfort.

You know as well as I that this life we have is but one and we are on a journey and it isn't so much WHAT we do as WHO we do it with—My Sunday school teacher last week asked—What is God teaching you right now? Then he said...if you say nothing then he will keep giving it to you until you figure it out...I guess life is all about your relationship with God and his lessons. I thank you for the many lessons he is teaching me through so many of you... and I truly thank you greatly for walking beside us these past few months.

Cathy

Specific Prayers
1) Counts will be good for chemo on Wednesday
2) Treatment will not cause too much turmoil in her body
3) Treatment on Thursday will be without concern

4) Praise that this is the LAST TOUGH treatment
5) Praise that God had his hand on her body and poured into her his strength through blood regeneration
6) Praise for a gallant prayer army that he has chosen and blended together for the healing of Molly.

Cathy

Praise God where ever you are and whatever situation He has allowed you to be in...His glory will shine through!

To: Jan
From: Cathy
Sent: Monday, June 5
Subject: Reply to her above e-mail:

I was despairing...you nailed it! God used Oswald Chambers to try to override my emotions when he quoted Hebrews 13:5&6 for June 4th and 5th. God will never leave me or forsake me; the Lord is my helper I will not fear! And then coming home after reading your dear words—BE STILL...and know that I am God! Yeah, he's here.. and then he sends precious angels like you to give me proof! Truly you will never know...and you know the rest of that line.

Love you,
Cathy

To: Lynda
From: Cathy
Sent: Monday, June 5
Subject: Checking on you

OK I'm just checking on your next move. Need to know what to pray for. How was orientation? Did Rebekah meet some fun people? And how did you do? AND HOW ARE YOU? I figure I can just e-mail you and you can answer when you want to and not if you don't. But to me, there was or is something to be said for having a note to tell you that somebody is thinking about you and I am and I love you. As a mom, you have got one tough role… This deal isn't for wimps!

Cathy

To: Cathy
From: Lynda
Sent: Monday, June 5

Hey-We just got home from orientation. She was with friends so wasn't as boring. Got her registered for fall. Putting in port on Mon. and starting chemo on Mon. She will have 1 hour a day for 5 days, weekends off, 5 more days and then a week off. 2 on and 1 off. Isn't that what ya'll are doing? She wants to go to school she just doesn't know how she will react to her chemo. We will have this summer to test it out. She can take her chemo in Ft. Worth's Cook's Hospital if she doesn't react badly. I will go up there and be there when needed at first. How are you guys doing? Did Molly get to take her treatment or did she have to have a transfusion? Only 1 more left and then radiation? I am going to make it over there this week cause don't know when I can again. I love you.

Lynda

To: Cathy
From: Kay L
Sent: Monday, June 5
Subject: God is Sovereign

HE put those cells in her, both red and white and HE is sovereign and HE can make the count go up if it is in HIS plan. HE is SOV-

EREIGN! I am praying that HE chooses to make that white count go up. HE loves her so much, HE died for Molly.

Love,
Kay

To: Cathy
From Beth B
Sent: Tuesday, June 6
Subject: Heart Words

Cathy,

I don't have any wise words, just "heart" words. I am thinking about you, praying, feeling very small, but knowing that my prayers as well as countless others are being heard and lovingly answered by our precious Lord, who is loving you and Molly unfailingly. You are an amazing mom. Thank you for sharing your thoughts, your feelings, and your faith with all of us. Do not think that it is without purpose.

Love in Christ,
Beth

P.S. One of my favorite verses, especially when I am faced with "enemies," such as fear, doubt, and despair...anything that keeps me from being victorious in Him.

> I love you, O Lord, my strength. You are my Rock, my Fortress, and my Deliverer. My God is my Rock in whom I take refuge. He is my Shield, the Horn of my Salvation, my Stronghold. I call to the Lord, who is worthy of praise and I am saved from my enemies. Psalm 18:1–3

[Such a sweetheart...this is a mother of four...and a grand mom... just like so many of you; I know she relates to this like she would if it was one of her own children. These words are such a comfort]

To: Cathy
From: Susan I
Sent: Tuesday, June 6

Thanks for sharing that wonderful reminder that God is always able.

Love,
Susan

[A prayer warrior and friend from church]

To: Cathy
From: Kitty
Sent: Tuesday, June 6
Subject: Devotional

May the blood of Jesus course through the veins of Molly and restore her counts today. In the mighty Name of Jesus. Amen.

Streams in the Desert
Author: Mrs. Charles E. Cowman
Program Date: June 5th, 2000

> "Make thy petition deep" (Isaiah 7:11)
>
> Make thy petition deep, O heart of mine,
> Thy God can do much more
> Than thou canst ask;
> Launch out on the Divine,
> Draw from His love-filled store.
> Trust Him with everything;
> Begin today,
> And find the joy that comes
> When Jesus has His way!
> —Selected

We must keep on praying and waiting upon the Lord, until the sound of a mighty rain is heard. There is no reason why we should not ask for large things; and without doubt we shall get large things if we ask in faith, and have the courage to wait with patient perseverance upon Him, meantime doing those things which lie within our power to do.

We cannot create the wind or set it in motion, but we can set our sails to catch it when it comes; we cannot make the electricity, but we can stretch the wire along upon which it is to run and do its work; we cannot, in a word, control the Spirit, but we can so place ourselves before the Lord, and so do the things He has bidden us do, that we will come under the influence and power of His mighty breath.—Selected

"Cannot the same wonders be done now as of old? Where is the God of Elijah. He is waiting for Elijah to call on Him."

The greatest saints who ever lived, whether under the Old or New Dispensation, are on a level which is quite within our reach. The same forces of the spiritual world which were at their command, and the exertion of which made them such spiritual heroes, are open to us also. If we had the same faith, the same hope, the same love which they exhibited, we would achieve marvels as great as those which they achieved. A word of prayer in our mouths would be as potent to call down the gracious dews and melting fires of God's Spirit, as it was in Elijah's mouth to call down literal rain and fire, if we could only speak the word with that full assurance of faith wherewith he said it.—Dr. Goulburn, Dean of Norwich

From: Cathy
Sent: Wednesday, June 7
Subject: Do I really trust God?

Well, she made it! The magic # was 1,000 and she had 1,100... It was a barely but she made it! So, tomorrow we will finish out this week's treatment without being dependant on counts and continue with one final treatment on Monday, again not depending on counts because it is the least taxing of the treatments. Then we will be done with the chemo part, skip a week and then radiation will start. I prayed for a straight line and though we shuffled a few days, God maintained the time line and we will be finished on the original schedule (Monday). Dr. McClain is amazed and said today that she has handled this protocol so beautifully and that it is just short of being miraculous.

Miracles do still happen and her handling this is of no surprise knowing the prayers that have lifted her up. Each time we get a good report, we comment on God's blessings and the prayer support, so I suspect that all who have watched this have a pretty good idea that it is God who has been faithful in guiding our way and has given wisdom and courage to make bold decisions to those who have cared for her.

Let me note here that I am really on the fence of saying that Monday will be our last chemo. For what if... and then I have to look at it the other way and think I TRUST GOD. I am standing on the promise that if I ask for this protocol to be completed in the timely way it was planned and I ask it in the name of the Lord, it WILL be done. I can't be scared that it might not happen. For if it does, then my request was answered and if it doesn't, then God has another plan. The "what if's" are in God's hands, just like the rest of this journey has been.

> Psalm 52:9 I will praise you forever for what you have done; in your name I will hope, for your name is good. I will praise you in the presence of your saints.

I asked Dr. McClain after he had seen the way Molly has responded to this Stanford V protocol if TCH will consider it for Hodgkin's patients in the future. He said yes that they were now considering this protocol as an option. So not only has she weathered this well but she has opened a door for new Hodgkin's patients. They will be able take part in a protocol whose treatments are not so long and intense and yet have the same curable percentages. God is big and working in so many different directions with such a variety of effects on relationships and circumstances. What a great and mighty God we serve.

Thank you dearly,
Cathy

Specific Prayer Requests:

1) Just let Molly hang on through these next five days safely
2) No breaks, no complications
3) Praise for the counts being just enough to qualify for today's treatment
4) Wisdom and clarity for decisions to be made for the next weeks ahead

Praise God wherever you are and whatever situation He has allowed you to be in... His glory will shine through!

To: Cathy
From: LuAnn
Sent: Wednesday, June 7

Dear Molly and Cathy:

You will never know how your faith during Molly's illness has strengthened so many. Thank you for sharing your feelings and battles and allowing your friends to lift you in prayer. God is so good and you are a testimony to that fact. I came across this devotional today and found encouragement. I pray you find hope and courage in knowing that God and so many of your friends care so much for you.

A little girl's father had been seriously injured in an accident and was in the hospital. The little girl was anxious and worried at bedtime, so she asked her mother if she could sleep with her. In the darkness of the room, the little girl asked, "Mommy, is your face turned towards me?" Her mother responded, "Yes," and soon the mother could hear the rhythmic, peaceful breathing of a little girl asleep. Then, the mother quietly slipped from bed and went to the window. She looked to the sky and asked, "Father, is your face turned toward me?"

Sometimes, God seems so very near, but other times, we experience uncertainty and insecurity as we face challenges that sap our strength and test our faith. In times of trouble we are challenged to remember that the only true security is found in God through Jesus Christ. And how comforting it is to know that the Father's face is always turned toward us.

Gigi Graham Tchividjian (Billy Graham's daughter) wrote:

> Weave the unveiling fabric of God's word through your heart and mind. It will hold strong, even if the rest of life unravels. Thy word I have treasured in my heart. Psalm 119:11a

> Let us draw near with a sincere heart full of assurance of faith. Hebrew 11:22

Praying peace and healing for you,
Lou Ann

[Friend from bible study... our older daughters were friends in high school... this is a sweet story of comfort]

To: Cathy
From: Jan G
Sent: Thursday, June 8
Subject: Don't be afraid

> Do not be afraid Daniel. Since the first day you set your mind to gain understanding and to humble yourself before Me, your words were heard and I have come in response to them. Daniel 10:12–13

We must be prepared to wait on God's timing. His timing is precise; for He does things at the very time He has set. So take heart little one for the One you wait for will not disappoint you. He will never be even five minutes behind "the appointed time." It is your heavenly privilege to trust ALL your needs to His glorious riches!

Love,
Jan

To: Cathy
From: Rob
Sent: Thursday, June 8

Great news—she's nearly finished—Rob

To: Cathy
From: Debbie K
Sent: Thursday, June 8
Subject: Encouragement

Cathy, you are amazing! I really do eagerly await your weekly e-mails! I feel like I've finished Bible study each time I read one!

Praise God for all of the answered prayers and MIRACLES! I know you are a witness to each doctor you encounter! And I love that when Molly asked you to ask for intercessory prayer about the transfusion, He chose to encourage Molly with that answered prayer!

I am praying for you and your family. I pray that you continue to be blessed by, throughout, and uplifted by Him during this challenging time. I know that this has been a roller coaster ride for each of you, and being sixteen and female doesn't make for a cake walk, but I praise God and know that He has the perfect plan for each of us.

Love,
Debbie

[This is my no fluff friend...who sees things as they are and gives me the courage to stand up in the face of adversity. Her humor is a delight and she is truly an encourager.]

To: Cathy
From: Kay L
Sent: Thursday, June 8
Subject: God answers prayers

You, know Cathy, which ever way it goes, God has answered the prayers of the people. Remember HE has a plan and we don't know what it is and that is how HE answers our prayers, by being a bigger God than we can wrap our minds around. HIS plan is perfect. What a praise that is. We are a blessed people to know HIM and know HE is sovereign and HIS ways and thoughts are higher than ours.

Kay

To: Cathy
From: Bonnie
Sent: Thursday, June 8
Subject: Thank you

Cathy—Thank you for the many lessons He is teaching me through you, Molly and your lovely friends. I am praying for you daily. It is because of the emails I receive each day that I sometimes feel like I am right there beside you even though I am miles away. Here is a big hug.

I love you,
Bonnie

[I love this because this is my childhood friend who lives in College Station and it shows the impact that these responses have not just on me but on all who are reading them.]

From: Cathy
To: Kitty
Sent: Friday, June 09
Subject: Molly

I have had the sweetest, most encouraging e-mails sent in the last few weeks but this week particularly. Thank you! Each of you will never know the power of your words and your timing. Molly not only made it through this week of tough treatments but she has had energy, she sat out in the sun, she has been hanging with friends and has defied the odds of what this weeks activities should have done to her body. Maybe just being so close to the finish line has given her a benefit of mind over matter. Whatever it is, "GOD" and friends we are most grateful.

There are just some quiet times that knock you off your feet more than others and this morning was one of them. I was telling God how undeserving I was of the favor he has shown, the blessings he has so richly and tenderly given and most especially how undeserving I was of his not only ALLOWING his son to die on my behalf but SENDING him to do just that. I was overwhelmed by God's spirit of compassion and just down right love he has for me…and you too. I apologized to him for my occasional yielding to a dark and gloomy vignette of thoughts…And then it occurred to me that when thunderstorms come my way, I don't yield to them. They just encompass my surroundings for a while and then move on. Each storm moves at its own speed and no two storms are alike. But what they do have in common is they tend to isolate you and keep you tethered pretty much to one place (unless you really have to move and change locations) and that space is where you watch and listen. In this storm we have been watching and listening and God has been speaking through his word, through words of each of you, and the rains are clearing.

After I had been walking for a while this morning, I asked God to join me and truly I had not taken 5 steps when I looked down and saw this round piece which looked to be a penny. It had been run over, was weathered, the edges were ragged, and it had turned a dark color. You really could hardly recognize it. I picked it up for I knew under all that wear there was an imprint stating IN

GOD WE TRUST. I knew it because it was familiar to me, something I had grown up with, held in my hand, believed in and used. Here it is years later as a reminder! The declaration was there yet it was disguised. I am sure it wasn't noticed by many but it was there, right there in the middle of the street.

Hebrews 11:1. Faith is being sure of what we hope for and certain of what we do not see. It reminded me of the storm that had been brought to mind earlier. God's there. When it is dark and gloomy and you don't notice him, and your circumstances are all unfamiliar and disguised, he is there right there beside you. It is OKAY to yield to sad thoughts as long as you realize that God is sad with you. Remember that he sees the end of the storm and the sunshine that will come after the wind and the rains go away. That is when he gives us the greatest gift of all ..."HOPE." It is that hope that gives you strength to weather the Storm. For it is in God that we must trust.

Romans 12:12 Be joyful in hope, patient in affliction, faithful in prayer.

P.S. I did get out the copper cleaner to confirm that that piece was a penny and after a bunch of elbow grease it finally appeared. If your life has been covered with the grime of the world, remember that God knows what is under all the stuff and you are a true treasure in his eyes!

Cathy

Praise God wherever you are and whatever situation He has allowed you to be in...His glory will shine through!

To: Cathy
From: Vivian
Sent: Saturday, June 10

Dear Cathy, I am so glad Molly made it through this very tough week. All of you have been in my prayers. She is an amazing young girl! What a battle she has been through. I pray for continued strength for all of you. "I can do all things in Him who strengthens me." I love you sweetie! My thoughts are prayers are with you every day!

VIV

[My college friend who could make me laugh all through the day. She was the one I saw the first day after Molly and I had gone down for the CT scan. She was in the hospital waiting room because of a thyroid problem. It was good to see a friend in the midst of strangers. Just a reminder that even in unfamiliar territory God would send a familiar face... and that "sweetie" part; that is sooo part of her warm and wonderful personality.]

To: Cathy
From: Kristy
Sent: Saturday, June 10
Subject: Copper penny

Thank you for your email, sweet friend, and for your update on Molly. I hope you know what an impact your emails and your witness are to me and to so many others. God is using you "in such a powerful way." I've always heard that term but have never experienced it so clearly and so closely. Thank you for sharing your walk, your ever-growing faith, and your friendship.

Molly, you, and all your family continue to be in my daily prayers.

Much love, another tarnished, beaten up, but ever hopeful penny.

Kristy

[When Kristy would read these e-mails she always seemed to have a wit about her response... notice the last line.]

To: Cathy
From: Susan I

Sent: Saturday, June 10
Subject: Worst days are best

Cathy,

I've been keeping up with Molly's progress and am so encouraged by what God has done in her and for her. In and for all the Jodeit family, actually. I'd like to share a quote from Charles Spurgeon that has always been an encouragement to me and I hope will be to you as well.

> I bear my witness that the worst days I have ever had have turned out to be my best days. And when God has seemed most cruel to me, He has then been most kind. If there is anything in this world for which I would bless Him more than for anything else, it is for pain and affliction. I am sure that in these things the richest, most tender love has been manifested to me. Our Father's wagons rumble most heavily when they are bringing us the richest freight of the bullion of his grace. Love letters from heaven are often sent in black-edged envelopes. The cloud that is black with horror is big with mercy. Fear not the storm. It brings healing in its wings, and when Jesus is with you in the vessel, the tempest only hastens the ship to its desired haven.

May our Lord continue to manifest His mercy, strength grace and love to you and your family.

Love,
Susan

[Wisdom at its best... worst days end up being the best]

To: Cathy
From: Lynda
Sent: Sunday, June 11
Subject: Bracelets

Thank you, thank you, and thank you! Did Molly get her chemo Wed? We missed YOU at Gina's. You're right. I'm not hanging: He's holding. LOVED, LOVED, LOVED our bracelets! Will wear them tomorrow! Any time things are said 3 times we should really pay attention! Jesus is HOLY, HOLY, HOLY!

luv ya,
lynda

[Week 12 of treatments...June 12]

To: Kitty
From: Cathy
Sent: Monday, June 12
Subject: Chemo Complete

SHE DID IT! She made it through the 12 week chemo timeline RIGHT ON TIME...and did it with flying colors. Her counts were low today but that didn't stop them from giving her treatment. She will have a transfusion tomorrow morning to give her a little boost. She is Okay with that. We will wade through this week called a chemo week and then a free week next week to give her body time to regroup a little. In 2 weeks from today she will start radiation. It is expected to be a 10 day treatment; 5 days for 2 weeks She will finish on July 7th and her 17th birthday will be on July 9th (a Sunday wouldn't you know it?). There is no way to thank you dear friends for the support through prayer that you have given her and all of our family but, here are the words please read between the lines—THANK YOU DEARLY AND SINCERELY—It is so apparent that she literally has been lifted to a level which is not and has not been comprehensible to many. For God has shown his hand in remarkable ways.

    I gave blood a couple of weeks ago as a backup if she needed it and that will be the blood she will use—(You can imagine the jokes already) She will only need one unit for now as a boost for the red blood cells. This is not an emergency, just a precaution to keep her out of danger. Jennifer (her oldest sister) will give blood within the next week or so just to have it on hand again and Jamie Ann (her other sister) is standing in the wait if we need more.

But these are the specific prayers for her for this week:
PRAISE: For the wonderful staff at TCH, for their true desire to make Molly comfortable and the encouragement and kindness they always extended to their patients
PRAISE: For the completion of the chemo cycle of this protocol and its effectiveness—(For her PET scan shows her to be completely clear)
PRAISE: For Dr. McClain and his honesty and intuitiveness and compassion for treating Molly. To him, each patient was individually assessed and a true desire to address their individual needs and anxieties were a priority to him. A true kind heart and gentle spirit.

Specific Prayers
1) MOLLY'S body ACCEPTS the blood without side effects including fever or rash
2) The doctors will talk tomorrow and decide the radiation plan—please pray for MINIMUM amounts TO PROVIDE HER SAFTEY in all areas
3) Please pray that if there are any lurking YOUNG OR OLD cancer cells hiding that they will be discovered and destroyed for LIFE AND AM I BOLD ENOUGH TO PRAY THAT THIS WILL BE THE ONLY INFUSION SHE WILL NEED... YOU BET!

Thank you,
Cathy

Praise God wherever you are and whatever situation He has allowed you to be in...His glory will shine through!

[The following e-mails are all in response to Molly completing chemo...this was a celebration not just for Molly but for all who have prayed her through it....for they too felt the joy of her victory through God's faithfulness. Most of the e-mails were sent in care of Kitty and she gathered them up and sent replies not only to me but the entire e-mail list was able to share the read.]

To: Cathy
From: Jan G
Sent: Monday, June 12

AND ALL GOD'S CHILDREN SAID...AMEN! OH HAPPY DAY! I LOVE YOU!

[This just makes you want to dance]

To: Cathy
From: Debbie K
Sent: Monday, June 12

Cathy,

I saw Molly last night at Molina's. She looks FANTASTIC! I told her that she should be the poster child for anyone who has been sick! No one looks that good even after they've been on vacation! I hope she feels as good as she looks! I did tell her that she's not going to get any sympathy looking like she does! She needs to mope around and milk this at home, anyway!

I pray that each of you can now relax and enjoy some free time for the next few days. And for the correct radiation dosages of every treatment to completely wipe out any residual cancer cells. And of course, that she handles the radiation even better than she did the chemo. We are all praying for you!

Debbie

To: Cathy
From: Carolyn F
Sent: Monday, June 12

Cathy, I read with ultimate joy your words of thanksgiving and praise for Molly's ending treatment today. There surely are angels surrounding the Jodeit family. I think of you both every day and I will continue to keep Molly (and you) in my daily prayers. God is good, indeed.

Love and hugs to all of you,
Carolyn

[This is my friend who finally could talk me into going to lunch... and believe me that isn't easy. You know how you have those really "safe" friends... she is one of mine!... and funny!!!! She can always make me laugh.]

To: Cathy
From: Allison
Sent: Monday, June 12

"Praise God for He is good, His faithfulness endures to all generations!" What a beautiful testimony this time has been to our gracious and loving and great God. I praise you, Lord, for walking Molly and her family through the shadows, for we know that shadows are only temporary and formed by a greater light above! I will be praying for all good results in the next treatments!

Love,
Allison

[Allison is one of Mary Leslie's wonderful friends who has stayed right with us on this journey... and is a friend now to us... I am always grateful for her encouragements... especially loved the shadow analogy]

To: Cathy
From: Kitty
Sent: Monday, June 12

Thank you, Cathy, for sharing your heart and letting your love and faith in our Lord Jesus shine through in this traumatic time. You have certainly lifted me up. Please God from Whom all blessings.

Kitty

[What a steady support and encourager Kitty has been through all of this]

To: Cathy
From: Audrey
Sent: Monday, June 12

Cathy, What a difficult though amazing journey you all have and are taking, yet continually being obedient in the next thing and walking right in our Lord's footsteps as he leads the way. Thank you for your willingness and transparency in letting us trail along side you. So, so many have been touched deeply by your faith, strength, and eternal perspective. As you once said, "the end of this story is not yet written," and I suspect God has a mighty work waiting for His precious Miss Molly. Praise God for this wonderful news!

Audrey

[Gentle spirited and strong in faith... in bible study and a sweet friend from our daughter Jamie's high school days]

To: Cathy
From: Lou Ann
Sent: Monday, June 12

God puts us all in each other's lives to impact one another in some way. Today we have all seen God's power and glory through what He has done for Molly. We are all awed by His provision and peace that has kept you strong.

The best and most beautiful things cannot be seen or touched—they mustbe felt with the heart—Helen Keller

I rejoice with you as only the heart of another mother can at God's provision for your child.

Happy moments, praise God.
Difficult moments, seek God.
Quiet moments, worship God.
Painful moments, trust God.
Every moment, thank God
Praising God for this immeasurable blessing

[She always found these little treasures to send back...I loved them]

To: Cathy
From: Dianne
Sent: Tuesday, June 13

Cathy, thank you for allowing the Lord to increase my faith by watching you boldly walk in faith. You have not been afraid to ask really big things of God because you know He can do all things. At the same time that you have boldly come to his throne you have been totally accepting of His will; for He has shown you that his love for Molly is deeper than we can begin to imagine. I am always going to remember how you demonstrated faith, asking for what we want and at the same time knowing that God hears our prayers and that He absolutely knows what is best!

I give Him praise and glory and honor. He is able to do exceedingly more than we can imagine. THANKS BE TO GOD FOR MOLLY'S RESULTS! It is such a privilege to bring Molly and your family before the Lord each day. What a blessing to see God's hand. My heart is overflowing with joy!

Dianne

[One of my Volleyball bleacher friends when Molly was in middle school...an Alabama sweetheart]

To: Cathy
From: Beth R
Sent: Tuesday, June 13

Cathy,

I have followed carefully the reports, the prayers, the thoughts—from you, Kitty, and so many others. A prayerful time, a horrible time, a blessed time. You and Molly are a constant inspiration to all. The Lord is truly with you two. He always is with us, but sometimes less visible. May His Light continue to shine upon you.

Much love,
Beth

[This is my sister by marriage… and was glad that she was able to follow us through this journey… for she was the liaison to her family and as well as an encouragement to me. She was and still is the family squire!]

[The following e-mail was sent to me by my friend Ruth Ann. She and her husband Ken have each treaded through the halls of cancer. Ruth Ann had breast cancer, Ken had Leukemia… and complications to follow. They are such ambassadors of Christ as they work through each day. Mel and I have watched as they have displayed their faith gallantly through continued adversity. These are some of the people who you learn great lessons by HOW they live as well as WHAT they say; their encouragement and wisdom have been beacons of light to help us tread through this journey of ours. For their ROCK is our Almighty God and it is on his foundation that they stand.]

To: Cathy
From: Ruth Ann
Sent: Tuesday, June 13

Praise God for the testimony of His grace, strength, and love through you during this entire journey and know that He is already in the next step even as you begin to lift your foot and move in oneness with Him. The time of radiation was such a peaceful and supernatural time for me as I knew I was resting totally in His arms. He gives the same assurance to Molly and His arms are so secure and warm and loving and safe and healing! Step by step with Jesus.

Much love, Ruth Ann

To: Cathy
From: Kitty
Sent: Wednesday, June 14
Subject: Faith

Title: *Watch Well Their Faith*
Book: Streams in the Desert Author: Mrs. Charles E. Cowman
Program Date: June 14th, 2000

"I have prayed that your own faith may not fail" (Luke 22:32).

Christian, take good care of thy faith, for recollect that faith is the only means whereby thou canst obtain blessings. Prayer cannot draw down answers from God's throne except it be the earnest prayer of the man who believes.
 Faith is the telegraphic wire which links earth to Heaven, on which God's messages of love fly so fast that before we call He answers, and while we are yet speaking He hears us. But if that telegraphic wire of faith be snapped, how can we obtain the promise?
 Am I in trouble? I can obtain help for trouble by faith. Am I beaten about by the enemy? My soul on her dear Refuge leans by faith.
 But take faith away, and then in vain I call to God. There is no other road betwixt my soul and Heaven. Blockade the road, and how can I communicate with the Great King?
 Faith links me with Divinity. Faith clothes me with the power of Jehovah. Faith insures every attribute of God in my defense. It helps me to defy the hosts of hell. It makes me march triumphant over the necks of my enemies. But without faith how can I receive anything from the Lord?

Oh, then, Christian, watch well thy faith. "If thou canst believe, all things are possible to him that believeth."—C. H. Spurgeon

We boast of being so practical a people that we want to have a surer thing than faith. But did not Paul say that the promise was, by FAITH that it might be SURE? (Romans 4:16)—Dan Crawford.

Faith honors God; God honors faith.

Phase II: On to Radiation

The following e-mail was sent to Dr. Link because Mel and I were just making sure we were doing our homework. I think I also had read too many confusing comments on the Internet. Dr. Link was a straight shooter when we first began this journey and he and Mel talked on the phone as soon as we had made the decision to go with the Stanford V protocol.

Dr. Link is Chief of Oncology at the Stanford University School of Medicine. We knew his experience was vast with this protocol. The many Hodgkin's cases that he has seen through his Stanford Hospital experiences would be an asset in settling our apprehensions about the radiation that Molly was going to have to endure.

We spoke to him at the beginning of this journey and here we are turning to him once again for confirmation. We wanted to be prepared and have learned over the past few months, that for Molly and all of us, it was better to be properly informed of what was to come. The fear of the unknown can take you down a pretty scary road.

The more we were informed (with basic information)...the more at ease we were...because so many times our thoughts ran amuck just because we had no idea of what to expect.

To: Dr. Link
From: Cathy
Sent: Wednesday, June 14

Dr. Link,

I have not met you but my husband, Mel Jodeit, spoke to you on the phone in late March (while you were at an Oncology Conference in Chicago) when our 16 year old daughter Molly was diagnosed by Dr. Ken McClain with Hodgkin's 4A. (Your name was given to us by Rob Ladd whose sister is a Dr. at Stanford and operated on your daughter's foot.) You were very encouraging when we came to you asking about the Stanford V protocol and there is where we decided to hang our hat. We have now completed the chemo phase and will be talking with Dr. Paulino (formerly with St. Jude's) in the next week or so regarding radiation. Since this regimen is so new to Texas Children's I just would like you to tell me your experiences with the radiation on this protocol. Molly's first follow up PET Scan was clear except for a blotch still in her neck and she was called an early responder—the follow up CT scan showed 50 to 70 % improvement in lymph nodes - most recent PET scan shows completely clear and the lymph notes are still slightly enlarged and they can't seem to get a good measure on them from the CT scan.

I have read enough to be so tentative about radiation and the long term effects yet I know this protocol requires radiation—you all seem to have done quite a bit of tweaking to give the least yet most effective combination of chemo drugs to achieve a 90% cure rate and I am just wondering what has been revealed about the need for radiation... the amounts, the specific fields, the protection, secondary cancers etc. Molly reacted amazingly to the chemo for 12 weeks... she made it from start to finish with just a two day delay in the last week but still ending on the scheduled time. We had an infusion on Tuesday because her hemoglobin was 7 but even that went so smoothly. She has maintained energy, great attitude, and has not taken on that chemo look—Dr. McClain has been absolutely terrific, honest, compassionate and quite frankly also amazed by the way she has weathered this protocol.

I know how busy you are and I appreciate so much your taking the time to read this—You all have done an outstanding job in research for Hodgkin's and we are ever so grateful that we were able to come on board with this regimen and that you all have been willing to share so freely all that you have learned—This radiation is new territory to us and I once again just need to hear from you some of your experiences or thoughts about the ways you have handled the road map for previous patients. I just think you all are on the cutting edge of treating this disease and if there have been any improvements or changes in the last months or years I would like to read about them.

Thank you again for your time,
Cathy Jodeit
Molly's mom

Praise God where ever you are and whatever situation He has allowed you to be in... His glory will shine through!

To: Cathy
From: Dr. Link
Sent: Wednesday, June 14

This is a bit complicated to handle via e-mail. I would appreciate if you would call my office and have me paged so we can talk about this. (It's easier to talk than to type!)

Michael P. Link, MD
The Lydia J. Lee Professor of Pediatrics
Chief, Division of Hematology/Oncology
Stanford University School of Medicine

[We did talk at great length on the phone. He gave me a heads up on many accounts and with that information I was able to ask appropriate questions and we were able to discern the validity of the procedures.]

To: Lynda
From: Cathy
Sent: Monday, June 12
Subject: Thinking about you

I thought about you the whole day... we are ending chemo the day that you are starting AGAIN! Don't you think that is a little weird? Hope it went ok—We are at Methodist tomorrow getting a transfusion; blood count was too low for her to be able to stay out of danger for radiation. We will start radiation 2 weeks from today. Can you even believe that we are talking about this? I'll be thinking about you tomorrow too! Please never feel the need to respond to my e-mails. I just know how much it helps me when I read that someone is thinking about us, and I want you to know that I am always thinking about you... and a live personal note always beats a forward... hands down!

Love you,
Cathy.

To: Cathy
From: Lynda
Sent: Wednesday, June 14
Subject: Response

You always make me laugh. Can you JUST give me a schedule you ask! YES I can JUST give you a schedule.

We go for one hour M-F for 2 weeks and then get a week off. We went this week and will go next week and then we will get a week off. No radiation.

I very rarely get out. Only to take her. I don't cook, I don't take or pick up the laundry very often, and I don't go to the grocery store. I sleep a lot and I think that that is my escape. We did take her and 8 of her friends to the ranch all last weekend. I just want her to be well and that pretty much covers it. I am pretty much resting and waiting on Him. He has and continues to meet all our needs. I've asked for about everything I can ask for so now I have the privilege of just praising Him and waiting on Him.

She is starting to have her friends take her now that it is down to an hour next week. I should have more time to myself. I would love to come over or go out. What are your radiation times? I was thinking about going to Ft. Worth this weekend and staying at David, Jr.'s house. He won't be there and when I get away like that it is really good for me. Then I thought I'll get there and probably miss my family plus it's Father's Day so I decided not to go. We want to go eat with you guys soon. You are truly a very important blessing in my life.

I love you,
Lynda

[She makes me laugh]

To: Cathy
From: Jill
Sent: Wednesday, June 14
Subject: Authority of God

> Now unto Him who is able to keep Molly without stumbling, slipping or falling, and to present her unblemished, blameless and faultless before the presence of His glory in triumphant joy and exultation with unspeakable, ecstatic delight——to the one only God, our savior through Jesus Christ our Lord be glory (splendor), majesty, might, dominion, power and authority, before all time and now and forever (unto all ages of eternity) Amen. (So be it) Jude 24–25

Amplified to God be the glory—great things He hath done!

Jill

[Spoken with such authority...by such a tiny little friend....shows you how big God is inside of her)]

To: Cathy
From: Claudia
Sent: Wednesday, June 14

I know you get a million of these but just to let you know I think and pray for you and Molly constantly. I love both you to pieces.

Claudia

To: Kitty
From: Cathy
Sent: Friday, June 16
Subject: Molly's Radiation Road Map

I was walking the other day on Chimney Rock and there was a lull on both sides of the street with traffic so I crossed while things were slow. When I got to the intersection there was a bunch going on and it was very congested. I was so thankful to already be on my side of the street.

As it is with prayer...Pray when things are quiet because you never know when life might get congested and you'll be glad you are already on the right side. Yesterday, we found out that the radiation part of Molly's treatment has taken a very different path than what we had expected. It is more intensive (dosage) than we first thought and much longer (time wise).

We are still whirling from initial information and are trying to get an immediate appointment with the designated radiologist, Dr. Paulino at Methodist who specializes in Pediatric Radiology. A patient is considered pediatric up until the age of 18 and in some cases 21. We did finish the chemo with flying colors. I know it was because of prayers, please hang with us for PART II. My friend Jeanne Frazier was sharing a story in Bible Study yesterday about being scared about reoccurrence of cancer and she said that she finally just dealt with the fact that "God would still be there." As he was the first time, he will be there still. I can't get that phrase out of my heart. "God is still there" Though this news is disappointing, GOD IS STILL THERE; GOD IS STILL HERE! He hasn't gone anywhere and just because circumstances have changed, HE HASN'T CHANGED Malachi 3:6 "I the Lord do not change."

Specific Prayer Request:
1) Open Dr. Paulino's heart to not just go by the book but look at Molly's case as an individual case and make decisions specifically designed to radiate only what needs to be radiated and only the amounts really needed to facilitate an extra arm of security for her cancer free body
2) Pray for our meeting on Monday at 1:30 with Dr. Paulino and Molly and Mel and I (This appt. just happened while writing this e-mail so God is already showing he has gone before us)
3) No more surprises—just to stay on track
4) We are taking Molly to LA to congratulate her for a hard fought battle. It is scheduled for Aug 2–6. Reservations have been made and we sure would love to make that deadline. Cancer free/treatment free/PICC line free
5) Pray for Molly to be able to hang on with a tenacious attitude and not be discouraged and shield her from fear and frustration of this unknown radiation territory
6) For the insurance company to respond in prompt way—for immediate treatment depends on their cooperation

Thank you so much,
Cathy

Praise God wherever you are and whatever situation He has allowed you to be in… His glory will shine through!

To: Cathy
From: Judy J
Sent: Friday, June 16

Cathy, as I saw you walking down the street Wednesday on your way home, I knew you were in conversation with God. I love that you are talking to him just as friends do walking in the neighborhood in the morning. Wait, you *were* walking with your friend in the neighborhood? When I saw you put on your tennis shoes and head out the door, I knew something wonderful was going to be revealed to you on your walk. What a walk! All your walks. We love to hear what is revealed to you. We are all walking with you. You, Molly and Mel and your entire family are so strong and I would never think of letting you down by forgetting to keep you in my prayers! You ALL are there. I think about you constantly and shoot little arrow prayers every time you come to mind. God cannot possibly move fast enough to miss those arrows! They are flying from all of us all the time. Monday will be good.

Love you,
Judy

[Tender hearted bible study friend…I love the comment about arrow prayers]

To: Cathy
From: Jan G
Sent: Friday, June 16

"When you walk, your steps will not be hampered; when you run, you will not stumble." Proverbs 4:12 We sit and weep in vain when the voice of the Almighty tells us to never stop moving upward and onward. Let us advance boldly whether it is dark and we can barely see the forest in front of us, or our road leads us through the mountain pass, where from any vantage point we can only see a few steps

ahead. Press on! It is such a comfort to drop the entanglements and perplexities of life into God's hands and leave them there.
Love,
Jan

[Always as if God were right in front of me speaking... I listened with great intent]

[I am including this e-mail to Jan because I want you, the reader to realize that things in my heart were not always quiet and positive. I had to fight through stuff just like everyone else does. I tried as often as I could to circumvent them but sometimes they literally just got the "best" of me... and I needed some strong Godly medicine to cure them. This was an example of one of those times!]

To: Jan
From: Cathy
Sent: Friday, June 16

You really are a messenger of our Lord God Almighty. I am running and asking God to not let me stumble... and talking about weeping—Jan I can't stop. I just hate this for Molly... I just keep thinking I am 53 and have never had to fight a battle such as this... I think of what her heart must feel like when she is all alone in the privacy of her room. I am just sick at my stomach! I just wish it were me. I am bigger and have more life tools! I just keep thinking she is only 16! I know we will get through this I know she will and we will be better for it... it is just hell seeing your precious daughter have to grow up this quick. Sometimes I think, no I know, that she is stronger than I am. It's God's grace in her that is bountiful. I am truly grateful for that and thank Him for that each day. What a blessing that he is actually riding her through this on his shoulders. OK, thank you once again for listening... no sleep... has caught up with me!

Love you,
Cathy

To: Cathy
From: Jan
Sent: Friday, June 16

My sweet, sweet precious friend—I cannot express strongly enough that when I read this, it is as if I were writing it! This is exactly what I would be saying and feeling and praying that I would be able to take this burden from my child. It is just incomprehensible that your baby is experiencing such a dramatic event when you are so willing to take it upon yourself. If only God's thoughts and ways were ours we could make it a perfect world for our children. There simply are no answers in our economy. I just keep hearing that still, small voice that says: "Little one, it is My thoughts, not yours. It is My way, not yours. I am the Great I Am. I am the Great Physician. Only trust and obey. Keep the faith that you so boldly share. Keep your eyes fixed on My Word, not your circumstances. I have brought Molly to this, and I will see My precious child through this. She is mine! Great things I have ordained for her and this is just a part of her journey. It is only for a while. Watch and wait and I will show you things that are beyond your wildest imaging's. Rest in My peace and know that know that you know that I am in complete control! Do you not know that when she is in her room she is not ALONE!!!! I am holding her in the palm of My hand and comforting her with My love, with my grace and with My Word. She is stronger that you think! Do not be afraid or anxious for anything. I am ALWAYS with her."

I love you beyond words,
Jan

To: Cathy
From: Georgiana
Sent: Sunday, June 18

I will be thinking about you all tomorrow. I just keep thinking about my friend's sister who went through this same illness many years ago and grew up to be an oncologist. We just can't see the whole picture now.

Love,
Georgiana

To: Cathy
From: Jane
Sent: Sunday, June 18

Dear Cathy,
I DO believe that Part I was such a success because God is listening to all the many prayers on Molly's behalf. I just know that Part II will be the same. I'm praying, praying. Bless Molly's sweet heart for being such a good patient and a fighter to lick this disease. Your reports each week have certainly been a blessing to me and I know to countless others. Your faith just warms my soul. God Bless you all.

Jane

[Sweet bible study friend... she is right, God is listening]

[Monday June 19—Radiation Consultation Meeting
Tuesday June 20—Molly went in to establish what is called a model
Thursday June 22–Radiation treatments began... total of 24 treatments; 8 upper fields and 8 lower fields, and then the 4 additional on spleen and 4 additional on neck.
We will start with upper and have two treatments completed this week! A week between upper and lower fields will be required for her body to have a chance to regroup.]

To: Kitty
From: Cathy
Sent: Monday, June 19
Subject: Molly begins Part 2 of her journey; radiation

And here we are in the showers of God's grace...I didn't have a chance to read Oswald Chambers yesterday so I picked it up first thing this morning and wouldn't you know that God waited for me to read it today for this would be so significant for the decisions of this day. I just love Peter and his relationship with God. I relate to him so often when he blunders. Today the title is "Keep Recognizing Jesus" and I won't track it all, but there are just a couple of comments that stood boldly in my face: Remember the story of Peter walking on water, Matthew 14 -the winds were big and the waves were high. When we evaluate Molly, our decisions for her are big and the stakes are high. PETER didn't consider them at all; he simply recognized the Lord, stepped out in recognition of Him and "walked on the water." THEN he began to take those things around him into account, and instantly down he went.

I have done such homework before this radiation meeting and I have been weary with circumstances. We hold such responsibility as we as parents have to step up to the plate and make hard decisions for the welfare of our children. This morning it just hit me hard that it holds greater responsibility for God to step in place for the responsibility of each of us...FOR GOD IS GOOD AND HIS LOVE ENDURES FOREVER. He has a bunch to live up to, AND A LOT MORE AT STAKE—HIS WORD.
SO THIS IS THE DEAL THAT I AM STANDING ON THIS MORNING...I will let my (Molly's) circumstances be what they may (like I have any choice)...but I will keep recognizing Jesus, and maintain COMPLETE reliance upon him— (Oswald Chambers) for we can make suggestions and make a case based on facts read but in the end it is God who has the final say...on decisions for Molly. He is Good and he will protect her and heal her HIS WAY.

I praise God for His mighty way and His love that strengthens us when we are weary.

I praise God for not just being a starter but a finisher
I praise God for His wisdom
I praise God that our ways are not His ways
I praise God that no concern is too small and insignificant for His involvement
I praise God that He can and will walk boldly through the fog of my thoughts and bring peace and calmness to my anxious heart
I praise God for biblical characters like Peter...

Prayer:
Thank you, Lord, for your loving kindness. Amen

The comments from Oswald Chambers are from his devotional book called My Utmost for His Highest.

Cathy

Praise God wherever you are and whatever situation He has allowed you to be in... His glory will shine through!

To: Cathy
From: Susan K
Sent: Monday, June 20

Cathy,

I can't tell you how inspirational you have been to me over the past 12 weeks. I have printed most of them out to just have and reread when needed. My family has prayed for you all and it has been such a joy to see the great reports that just keep coming. I have learned so much from all of you throughout this journey. I love your attitude, your gratitude and your faithfulness throughout all of this and I am truly amazed by your strength and your trust in the Lord. When I see the emails from Kitty I am always excited to open them knowing that I am going to once again experience something special when I read them. I wish I knew Molly but from all I have read, I do know that she is an amazing young woman who is so strong and full of hope and loved by so many. She is what the

Lord wants us all to be like. I am so happy for all of you that the chemo is over and will continue to pray for her full recovery. I hope the radiation treatments go well and over quickly. I would be happy to give blood if ever needed. I am a type O positive and Larry is O negative. Thank you so much for sharing with all of us and teaching us through your faith and your knowledge. It has truly been a gift.

Many blessings to all of you,
Susan

Sent June 20 from Rob:
Just checking to see how you were holding up! Rob

[A terrific friend and former boss]

To: Kitty
From: Cathy
Sent: Friday, June 23
Subject: Radiation Begins Next Week

I have so many different thoughts in my head and have been bombarded by restlessness and inadequacy all week. Then my sweet friend, Helene, called this morning and something clicked and reminded me that Satan knows where the cracks of my heart are. He knows just how and when to slither in and pounce. In the many prayers I have lifted up to God I had forgotten to ask him to give me a shield of protection from Satan...I had let it slip. Then it occurred to me; if these e-mails are in fact making a difference to some then he (Satan) is going to do whatever he can to derail them and he did just that this week. I couldn't get anything in writing because he was messing with my thoughts and emotions. Shows you how easily Satan can paralyze you.

This week we had consultations on Monday for radiation. Molly had an initial appointment on Tuesday and the actual radiation began Thursday. We consulted with the team and told them of our plans to be out of here on August 2nd and yesterday wouldn't you know, the schedule is 12 week days on, July 4th excluded, a week off and then an additional 12 days on again. When you do the math, we are finished on Aug 1. The thing about praying for God's will is that when you do and you are "expecting" him to follow through then you start looking anxiously for his hand anywhere and in everything.

1) The schedule was vastly different than what we had originally been told. We were dealing with that and then it was slightly altered again and now it has potential of working; God's hand is upon us.
2) When we walked in the radiation lobby on Tuesday there was a dated flip book at the registration desk… Tuesday's read: Miracles still Happen, expect them…. God's hand again.
3) In the reception area there was a guest book where patients have written encouraging words to other patients… BIBLE— Basic Instructions Before we Leave Earth… (reminder to keep it close) God's hand
4) The sweetest nurse—of course I am crying in the room before the consultation even begins (emotions, don't know where they come from or when they are going to sprout) and Molly is just looking at me and slightly rolling her eyes (she is calm, cool and collected… nothing new)—the nurse says—you all are doing just exactly what each of you is suppose to do in the season that you are in–Molly, 16, is suppose to be looking at you like "oh no, not again." (Truly this child was the most precious, solid thinking, calm soul… you just can't believe how she has handled all of this up to now… and still she stands gentle and strong… I am so proud and honored to be her mom) You are the mom and you are suppose to be hurting and wanting more than anything to take your daughter's place… these are God's seasons… sweet and needed perspective from God's hand
5) Even this week I have seen Molly continue to grow stronger.. God's hand
6) Mel was out of town and when he came back Wednesday, he was there as the usual rock with wisdom, guidance and encouragement for me to have courage to stand up and speak about my concerns to the radiation medical team. He provided such strength

especially when I started growing weary. I just hated watching Molly have to endure this! God's hand

7) There is a strong Christian mom with a 16 year daughter who is Volleyball player from Richmond who is scheduled to be in the waiting room the same time that I am each day. What a blessing, especially today, to visit with someone who understands. God's hand

8) Today's treatment was much more efficient and honoring to Molly's comfort. God's hand.

I know God is with us. I know God has a plan. I know God will use this for his Glory. I know what I know, but I am so easily tilted when I see Molly struggle with any of this and it takes constant reminding that this too will pass. We have to look at the hurdles we have already jumped and made it over without falling, and this part too will be successful.

I think sometimes the hardest part of doing something new is not knowing what to expect. Now we have gotten over the NEW of this phase—so I expect the rest will just fall into line.

Specific Prayer Request:
1) ARMOR - Please pray that God will shield us and fill any unseen cracks in his protective wall
2) Molly's counts to stay steady. With radiation, as with chemo, the attacks not only kill the bad cells but they destroy some good ones too. Please protect her GOOD cells and let them be strong and keep her immunities, platelets, and hemoglobin in
good enough condition to make it through this process without interruption
3) HEAL HER FULLY AND COMPLETELY FOR HER LIFETIME
4) Precision for the radiologist as they control the emissions
5) That the machines would work without hesitation or delay
6) That God would comfort Molly with HIS thoughts and peace as she is having to be still day after day
7) To guard Molly's body against a serious sore throat, and any thyroid complication during these days or in the future.

Thank you for your continues prayers—they are of great comfort!

Love,
Cathy

Praise God wherever you are and whatever situation He has allowed you to be in...His glory will shine through!

To: Cathy
From: Kitty
Sent: Friday, June 23

Title: *Don't Look at the Waves*
Book: Streams in the Desert
Author: Mrs. Charles E. Cowman
Date: June 23

When Peter was come down out of the ship, he walked on the water, to go to Jesus. But when he saw the wind boisterous, he was afraid; and beginning to sink, he cried, saying, Lord, save me" (Matt. 14:29–30).

Peter had a little faith in the midst of his doubts, says Bunyan; and so with crying and coming he was brought to Christ. But here you see that sight was a hindrance; the waves were none of his business when once he had set out; all Peter had any concern with, was the pathway of light that came gleaming across the darkness from where Christ stood. If it was tenfold Egypt beyond that, Peter had no call to look and see.

When the Lord shall call to you over the waters, "Come," step gladly forth. Look not for a moment away from Him.

Not by measuring the waves can you prevail; not by gauging the wind will you grow strong; to scan the danger may be to fall before it; to pause at the difficulties, is to have them break above your head. Lift up your eyes unto the hills, and go forward—there is no other way.

> Dost thou fear to launch away?
> Faith lets go to swim!
> Never will He let thee go;
> 'Tis by trusting thou shalt know
> Fellowship with Him.

Kitty

To: Cathy
From: Kay L
Sent: Friday, June 23

Cathy,

Can you believe how sweet and caring all the people are in the radiation area? And there are Christians all around. I was so amazed. God will use you to encourage others along in their faith. If ever you come across some nurse or blood person or anyone that seems grumpy, ask them about themselves and they will begin to open up and you can then ask them how you can pray for them. God will use you in ways you will never know. And when you are caring for others, you won't think about yourself or your situation. Jesus will give you the words.

Love to you, Mel and Molly. I am so glad we have the pictures of all of you when you came to Jackson Hole. I love looking at that picture. Remind Molly of having coffee with Monroe and Sweetie early in the morning sitting in the window seat.

How is that precious grandbaby? I keep thinking of the lessons you are teaching by your actions to your other kiddos.

Love,
Kay

[She is a cancer survivor who has traveled many of our same roads... she was even at the same radiology area at Methodist Hospital]

To: Cathy
From: Beth R
Sent: Friday, June 23

Such a tough week. Sometimes the path is hard to find. But I think you all are back on track. The light of His Presence on all of you, not just Molly. God bless and keep all of you.

Many prayers and much love,
Beth

[I love the word light here, for that is what we needed to see]

To: Cathy
From: Helene
Sent: Saturday, June 24

This email, after our conversation yesterday, was one HUGE answer to prayer. Just when things seem the absolute worst and we are nearly ready to throw in the emotional towel, God knows we need a break and steps in and covers us with just what we need to bring us back. My heart feels so very FULL at this moment; full of the joy that comes from seeing God working, actually working. The Bible says that no one has "seen" the face of God. I respectfully disagree. I believe we see Him constantly. You saw Him yesterday and so did I... through your email.

Helene

[Helene had called yesterday when I just needed someone to talk to and someone to remind me that even though things may look a little dark... God is still there and in control... God used her to be his vessel... it truly is amazing how much a little word of encouragement can light up your life. God just knows!]

To: Cathy
From: Tom S
Sent: Sunday, June 25

Molly has the worst behind her... tell her we love her and our prayers are with all the Jodeit's, as you know. We really love the Jodeit family and want all to get back to normal and know that it will!

T

[I think this really struck a cord with Tommy's (my brother) family because of Molly and his girls being such close friends and so close in age... it was hard to believe and take in]

[Week 2 of radiation... Molly should have 7 treatments completed by weeks's end only 17 left after this week]

To: Kitty
From: Cathy
Sent: Monday, June 26
Subject: Don't Fear God is Near

Our little BATMAN friend—(you remember the one who wears the cape that has Fear No Evil—Psalm 23 embroidered on the bottom) has completed his chemo and will now follow us to radiation. He has had 49 infusions since he started this journey and he is only 7 and they have been dealing with his cancer since November. Talking about putting OUR BLESSINGS IN PERSPECTIVE... THEY HAVE A CLEAN REPORT FINALLY... and his dad today said the God who has healed this is the God who has the power to keep it forever gone... what a testimony.

    Made me think about my testimony and I hope this will make you think about yours. We all have been given different trials and adversities. Some are just huge and over the top and seem like they are going to last indefinitely. Some seem like they are just trickles that do just enough to frustrate us and make us anxious. Whatever yours is and you know mine; I have to ask myself the same question that was asked in church last Sunday, "Am I BOLD enough to DECLARE the workings of my Almighty God? Am I willing to use Excellent as one bookend and Able as the other as the binding characteristics of God?" Between the bookends is the STUFF that God has ordained to be Good in the end! I am a little wimpy about declaration. But as each day closes and the lights are dimmed, it is worthy to look up at the sky and Thank God and BOLDLY Declare His Mighty Acts of this very day... and then look forward to what he has planned for the next!

Day 3 of the first series of 12 radiation treatments was today—we are on a roll—even though the machines were down for 2 hours. When Molly finally went in she was only there for 15 minutes—and came out smiling. The treatment for this day was over! Her hemoglobin was higher than it has been in over 2 months and platelets were strong as well—Thank you God She needs some prayer help on the white blood cells. She is on low alert—not allowed to be around crowds at malls, church etc. because her immunities are down. God can/will handle that.

I will not share a day by day unless we have something specific (like the white blood cells) to request. Everybody has their own backpack of issues and I hopefully have not imposed ours on you, but each member of our family is so very grateful for your prayers and do not take for granted one moment the impact they have made. I pray for each of you and thank God for your lives and ask His hand of grace to gently rest upon you heart.

This is day that the LORD has made... we are rejoicing and are glad to be alive.

Specific Prayer:
May Molly's body replenish the needed white blood cells so that she may carry on with tenacity the job that has been set before her... TO GET WELL !

> Let them give thanks to the Lord for His Love and for
> the miracles he does for people... Psalm 107:8

Psalm 19:8–11
The ORDERS of the Lord are RIGHT; they make people HAPPY
The COMMANDS of the Lord are PURE; they LIGHT up the way.
RESPECT of the Lord is GOOD; it will last FOREVER
The JUDGEMENTS of the Lord are TRUE; they are completely RIGHT
They are worth more than gold even the purest gold.
They are sweeter than honey.
By them your servant is warned.
KEEPING them brings great REWARD

Lovingly,
Cathy

Praise God wherever you are and whatever situation He has allowed you to be in...His glory will shine through!

To: Cathy
From: Kitty
Sent: Tuesday, June 27
Subject: Devotional

Title: *The Lord is My Strength*
Book: Streams in the Desert
Author: Mrs. Charles E. Cowman
Program Date: June 27th, 2000

"The Lord hath sent strength for thee" (Ps. 68.28, PBV).

The Lord imparts unto us that primary strength of character which makes everything in life work with intensity and decision. We are "strengthened with might by His Spirit in the inner man." And the strength is continuous; reserves of power come to us which we cannot exhaust.

"As thy days, so shall thy strength be"—strength of will, strength of affection, strength of judgment, strength of ideals and achievement.

"The Lord is my strength" to go on. He gives us power to tread the dead level, to walk the long lane that seems never to have a turning, to go through those long reaches of life which afford no pleasant surprise, and which depress the spirits in the sameness of a terrible drudgery.

"The Lord is my strength" to go up. He is to me the power by which I can climb the Hill Difficulty and not be afraid.

"The Lord is my strength" to go down. It is when we leave the bracing heights, where the wind and the sun have been about us, and when we begin to come down the hill into closer and more sultry spheres, that the heart is apt to grow faint.

I heard a man say the other day concerning his growing physical frailty, "It is the coming down that tires me!"

"The Lord is my strength" to sit still. And how difficult is the attainment! Do we not often say to one another, in seasons when we are compelled to be quiet, "If only I could do something!"

When the child is ill, and the mother stands by in comparative impotence, how severe is the test! But to do nothing, just to sit still and wait, requires tremendous strength. "The Lord is my strength!" "Our sufficiency is of God." The Silver Lining.

To: Cathy
From: Jan
Sent: Thursday, June 29

I just love what Cathy wrote a few days ago and I quote: "we all have been given different trials and adversities. Some are just huge and over the top and seem like they are going to last indefinitely, some seem like they are just trickles that do just enough to frustrate us and make us anxious. But as each day closes and the lights are dimmed in the sky it is worthy to look up and thank God and BOLDLY DECLARE His mighty acts of just this day and then look forward to what He has planned for the next." I was reminded this morning that the peace of God is an eternal calm. Anyone who enters the presence of God becomes a partaker of that undisturbed calm. "The peace of God, which transcends all understanding, will guard your hearts and your minds in Christ Jesus." Philippians 4:7

Love,
Jan

[She thinks really so much like I do... so that is why she likes some of these e-mails so much... she relates so clearly to them.]

To: Kitty
From: Cathy
Sent: Friday, June 30
Subject: Birds

I had this vision the other day in my quiet time of a big, I mean huge (as large as an airplane), flying bird. He was black and scary and hovering right over Molly and me and because he was so big and hovering we couldn't see the landscape. Then in the blink of an eye, the bird was transformed into a bunch of tiny birds that were no longer hovering but flying carefree. I know this sounds weird, but I get these visuals in my head and to me they make so much sense.

For if you look at life, don't you sometimes feel that huge black bird hovering? It can mean anything; loneliness, finances, a broken relationship, a health issue, anything. As long as that bird is allowed to linger, it blurs out the good view, the beauty of life itself.

But we have a choice:
1) To let it linger or
2) To ask God to transform it into a bunch of little birds so that you are not imprisoned by the intimidation of something so huge.

This is kind of the way this cancer journey has been. It started out as a great big black bird hovering and scaring the tar out of us but, God has now transformed it into being a bunch of small battles that we can fight one at a time.

Mel bought me a bird feeder... we used to have it under a canopy of trees hanging low but we have moved it to a high branch. It now swings in the wind and the squirrels can't get to it. It is in front of my kitchen window and I can't tell you the number of times just watching these tiny birds (and blue jays and cardinals and woodpeckers, too) have truly dissolved anxious thoughts and been such a reminder of God's provision even for tiny birds.

> Matthew 6:25 Therefore I tell you, do not worry about your life, what you will eat or drink; or about your body, what you will wear. Is not life more important than food, and the body more important than clothes? Look at the birds of the air; they do not sow or reap or store away in barns, and yet your heavenly Father feeds them. Are you not much more valuable than they? Who of you by worrying can add a single hour to his life? And why do you worry about clothes?

I have a pillow in my bedroom that says "Each Bird thinks his own nest charming", I think God wants us to be content in our nest, and find it charming, even when storms come and the winds blow hard. For in that nest is not only you or I but a dearly devoted Father who has promised to be with us always.

Phillipians 4:11 I am not saying this because I am in need, for I have learned to be content whatever the circumstances.

My prayer for each of you today is that you be willing to ASK God to transform any of those Huge Black Birds that are hovering over you into gentle non threatening peaceful flyers. May they represent the strength our Almighty God has to turn the big things into little ones at the touch of His hand. May they also remind you of the Grace that God has chosen to pour into our lives when we have done nothing to deserve it!

With love—and a Happy and safe Fourth of July,
Cathy

Praise God wherever you are and whatever situation He has allowed you to be in...His glory will shine through!

[Week two of radiation; July fourth she will be off!]

To: Kitty
From: Cathy
Date: Sunday, July 2
Subject: Detours and Potholes of Radiation

Why is that people who have traveled down a road before us are so credible? I would bet that it is because they have seen some of the pitfalls, they relate to some of our emotions, they made it through their trial and they are able to provide a hope. They are familiar with the road. They can tell you where the construction barriers are, where the road gets really bumpy, what you might see along the journey and how to best navigate to the next rest spot.

We travel I-10 every day and one day when I was driving back from Katy, I looked around and thought I just can't figure out how this is all going to end up. There are overpasses everywhere and extensions and curves along the feeder roads, new exits and entrances and really it just looks like a huge mess. But then I realized that there is a master plan, and on that master plan everything makes sense. The detours and potholes and construction all will have made contributions to the finished freeway. It will take some time to make all the changes and adjustments, but in the end, all the mess will be gone and we will have the benefit of the toils of construction.

As it is with life, don't you think? Our lives and a construction job seem to have a lot in common. We have to make strategic decisions when we set out for improvement in our lives. There will be detours and potholes for sure, but God, the Master Planner, will take all these diversions and use them to build a stronger, less congested, simplified, peaceful, joyful life.

Think about the contributions that potholes and construction and detours in your life have made to who/what you are now. God has traveled the road before us...he is familiar with each of our personal journeys and is just waiting for us to come to Him for wisdom.

These last few months we have learned perseverance, courage, patience, and a real appreciation for God, our Master Planner. His ways are not our ways, and though from the outside things look askew, there is a plan in the workings that is being guided by his divine touch.

I do have a specific prayer for Molly:
She has to have 8 radiation treatments on upper body and 8 treatments on lower abdomen. There are 4 additional treatments to a specific upper spot on her neck and 4 additional treatments on a spot in her spleen. I have requested that Dr. Paulino combine those 2 treatments of 4 days thus decreasing her treatments by 4 days. This is huge because he said that that is not general procedure but he would take it into consideration and let me know next week. I asked him to please assess Molly's case as an individual one not one of general protocol; he has agreed.

The prayer: Combine the 4 day treatments if it is safe for her body. Please also pray that when we take blood counts tomorrow that she will show great improvement over this last week.

GOD IS ABLE TO DO EXCEEDINGLY MORE THAN WE CAN EVER IMAGINE…When someone asked how many more treatments Molly had; I answered 17! My friend Jane P… (when standing beside me before the church service) corrected me and said 13. DONE…I love having bold friends stand in my gap! I got off my fence and boldly accepted her confidence.

Thank you again tenderly and graciously for your continued prayers…we cherish them and cherish you. May God bless you with his blessings and may your eyes be open to see them and your ears to hear them.

Cathy

Praise God where ever you are and whatever situation He has allowed you to be in… His glory will shine through!

To: Cathy
From: Kathy O
Sent: Monday, July 3

You and your family are an inspiration to us all… your courage and faith lift me up each day. Cathy, you and Molly are in my daily prayers.

And I agree with Carolyn... your thoughts and prayers should be published... there is a universal thread that connects so many of us! Thank you so much for allowing me to be a part of your journey! God Bless!

Kathy O

[This is a friend who was in our bible study many years back, went to work and was no longer able to attend; she asked to stay on the e-mail list because even before this you could count on Kitty sending some great life application Christian E-mails]

To: Cathy
From: Brian and Leslie
Sent: Monday, July 3

Cathy,

You are so amazing and Brian and I were just talking about how blessed Molly is to have you and Mel. God's glory will shine through!! Cathy, when mom was sick last year she was amazing too with her faith! Everyday she did her little devotional and in her book she wrote the best she could the verse from Matt.6:33: "But seek first his kingdom and his righteousness, and all these things will be given to you as well. Sometime our anxious hearts get the best of us, but prayer can really calm that. You have probably already read this book, but if you haven't it is so great. It is called Calm My Anxious Heart by Linda Dillow. Let me know if you have it because if you don't I want to send it to you! I have been in San Antonio for 2 weeks helping Erin move into a house and we were just talking about Molly last week. I have just sent Erin and Julie your e-mails because I know what ya'll are going through has taught you lots of perseverance, patience, and courage, but your testimony speaks volumes!!! Hang in there and we will be praying for Molly, you, Mel, Molly's improvement and that her counts will be improved!! We love you guys!!

Brian and Leslie

The following quote was on my Google opening page one day.... each day Google randomly selects quotes and this was one of them. I knew nothing of this man just really liked the quote. Many months later Tom, my son brought his name, out of the blue, up at a family dinner. My interest was peaked. I found that he is a wonderful writer and a strong Christian man. He has a tremendous sense of humor and is known as one of the giants (no pun intended; he weighed over 300 pounds) of Christian writers. He is worth investigating.

To: Kitty
From: Cathy
Sent: Tuesday, July 4
Subject: Molly—good counts

I read this quote yesterday and something about it just stuck ...
"An adventure is only an inconvenience rightly considered. An inconvenience is an adventure wrongly considered."—G K Chesterton, English author & mystery novelist (1874—1936)
I love an adventure. This morning I grabbed the dogs for a walk. I knew the rain was coming but I thought we could make it back in time. I asked God to let us get around the block please before the rains fell. God answered, but not in the way I had requested. We had been out for only 10 minutes or so and the rains came down... and not just sprinkles! I remembered this quote from yesterday and thought this is an adventure. I haven't been caught in the rain in ages and now here I am with two labs (one being the puppy Bentley who is now a big teenager). We were drenched. The dogs were frolicking through the ditches and having a wonderful time and there was not much I could do except choose to enjoy the circumstances, and I did. It was as though we were all celebrating the day and it was truly fun. (If we would have waited just an hour we would have missed the moment because the sun came out) I thanked God that He did let it rain on us because He changed the everyday momentum into something new. Oh, how I wish I could do that more often. Not the rain thing necessarily but the momentum and the attitude.

For God sees joy in so much that we see drudgery in. And walking in the rain was just a reminder to change things up a little—don't be satisfied with the same ho- hum, do something/anything in a different way. It helps you to take a new picture of life... and you will find the joy that God has waiting.

> Psalm 28:7 The LORD is my strength and my shield; my heart trusts in him, and I am helped. My heart leaps for joy and I will give thanks to him in song.

Molly's counts came back yesterday and they are higher than they have been in weeks—(White, red and platelets) PRAISE GOD As far as the combining of the treatments—that is still up in the air but because her counts are good, there is a possibility that she will not have to skip a week between treatments and will be able to work straight through the 2 radiation schedules. Her taste buds are messed up—but her throat is still good so:

Prayer Request:
Praise God for good counts
Psalm 126:3 The LORD has done great things for us, and we are filled with joy.

Praise God for not dropping the ball and following this through until the end (I am such a starter and not a good finisher so this really is something that I cherish and admire)
Praise God that He kept Molly safe when counts were so very low
Protection of any further discomfort of mouth and throat area
That His timing shall be what is important... not ours!

Thank you, Hope you have had a good holiday,

Love,
Cathy

Praise God wherever you are and whatever situation He has allowed you to be in... His glory will shine through!

To: Kitty
From: Cathy
Sent: Wednesday, July 05
Subject: Dr. Paulino said YES

I just can't believe it but... Dr. Paulino said YES to our request to combine the 2, four day treatments. We have an appointment with him tomorrow and will find out about aborting the week to be skipped as well. We are so thankful (Molly and I)! This cuts off almost a week and we can so see the end. Eleven more treatments; eleven days. We have taken this project and step by step adjusted to the requirements that have been made. God and his mighty hand have shown His favor over and over to Molly. It has to be through your fervent prayers! There are no words to say thank you. We have prayed for friends we know of and the friends who have prayed on our behalf who we don't know. We have asked God to show His favor upon you as well. You have been diligent and great warriors in a mighty battle. May you each be blessed.

Life throws us some curves! And sometimes when they hit we end up in a small bunker. We need a hand to help pull us out. Sometimes we land in a pretty dark and deep pit barely able to see light and we need more than a helping hand. When you are in that pit maybe it would help to imagine it this way... Dark pit no way out. So God comes down there with you so you at least will have a little company. Usually you have to ask Him because He wants to know that you want Him there. It might seem like forever before you start to see any signs of God doing anything to help the situation (you have to be willing to accept His help) then He carves out... THE STEP OF COURAGE... It's just one little step. It's not going to get you too far but at least it's a step. (You know when you are climbing up out of the swimming pool in the deep end and there are steps but they are not much good without the handrail) Well, with these steps, take each one as they come and let GOD be your HANDRAIL!

  FIRST STEP IS COURAGE
  THEN PERSERVERANCE
  THEN FAITH

THEN WISDOM,
THEN PATIENCE,
THEN TRUST
REPEAT AND REPEAT AGAIN UNTIL YOU
FINALLY YOU HAVE REACHED THE TOP
THAT TOP AND FINAL STEP HAS THE
GLORY OF GOD WRITTEN ALL OVER IT!

For He was there with you at the bottom and will be your handrail to the top!

Psalm 37:23 If the LORD delights in a man's way, he makes his steps firm;

Proverbs 16:9 In his heart a man plans his course, but the LORD determines his steps.

Galatians 5:25 Since we live by the Spirit, let us keep in step with the Spirit.

Jeremiah 12:23 [Jeremiah's Prayer] I know, O LORD, that a man's life is not his own; it is not for man to direct his steps.

Once you get out of that pit, you will KNOW what to do when the next curve ball comes...Duck!...If it comes so fast that it hits, remember to ask God to come be with you and carve out your first step. You have already seen the Hand of God and His glorious blessings! Remember, just one step at a time...

Cathy

Praise God wherever you are and whatever situation He has allowed you to be in...His glory will shine through!

To: Cathy
From: Vivian
Sent: Thursday, July 6

Oh Cathy, Praise God! Cathy, your words are so beautiful. Thank you for sharing your "battle" with us and your strong faith. I love you, honey, and pray for you and your sweet Molly all the time. (So do my family and friends) Give Molly my love.

Love,
Vivian

[Notice the "honey"... you would love her if you met her... sweet, warm, happy, funny...]

To: Cathy
From: Debbie K
Sent: Thursday, July 6

I am happy for Molly and you! Keep being her advocate with the Dr.'s; I think another idea is such a good thing! And your words are powerful, your imagery is perfect! I'm praying for continued and complete healing! Love you guys!

DK

To: Cathy
From: Terri
Sent: Thursday, July 6

Cathy, We are truly blessed that our paths crossed with your family as well—I know our Lord Jesus has his hand upon Molly and Kristin because he formed them in our womb and created them for great and mighty things- Remember they are fearfully and wonderfully made! (Psalm 139) They have already touched so many by their courage and faith and strength.

Love,
Terri

[This is my new friend who also had a 16 year old daughter going through radiation at the same time we were.... she was such a blessing who God had sent to me. She would only be there for the first couple of weeks but her faith was so strong and she so witnessed to me... How is it that God can follow through with details such as these... and get the timing right and the personalities right and the place right? Because he's God... that's how!]

To: Cathy
From: Kay L
Sent: Thursday, July 6

Cathy, once again the sermon Sunday up here in the Jackson church was "finishing strong" And you send this in your email.... God is amazing the way He shrinks distance and allows us to hear Him say the same thing different times and places to confirm He is sovereign. Praising God for the good counts.

Love,
Kay

To: Cathy
From: Pam
Sent: Thursday, July 6

YES...YES...YES... A million praises to God and His hand of mercy and grace.

[Pam is my son-in-law Blake's mom... a wonderful cheerleader and new friend from Dallas]

[She has completed 11 treatments... all of upper field and three of the lower field.]

To: Kitty
From: Cathy
Sent: Friday, July 07
Subject: Molly's Is an Intern

Molly continues to be strong—and just so you will see the whole picture right now—she interviewed for an internship at a cosmetic company on Wednesday.

Note here: Remember at the very beginning of this journey when Dr. Muntz told Molly he knew someone who owned a cosmetic company and if she would send him her resume; he would make a call... well she did and he did!

She started work yesterday (Thursday) at their distribution center in Stafford.

We go to Methodist each morning and she will go to work from 12:00—4:00 each afternoon for the month of July. Amazing that her tall lean body has been so strong and she is able and willing to do this. It reminds me that God is interested in the All of us not just the physical, or mental or spiritual but the ALL of us. She has been battling physically for months but this gives her a chance to get back into thinking outside that cancer box. I will say that she has continued to be able to do that each time we leave a treatment of any kind. It is over and... she turns it off.

This internship is such a positive adventure for her. She has a tremendous flare for fashion and this gives her a chance to see the behind the scenes workings of cosmetic business... Goes back to that adventure thing!

I thought about God being interested in the ALL of us and it reminded me of that wonderful potter example about God being the Potter and you being the clay. God is busy shaping us for his glory. Clay can't shape itself—we need a potter.

This is an excerpt from Oswald Chamber "My Utmost for his Highest" July 6)... I just love the way he puts things into focus!

Ever since God gave us the vision, He has been at work.

He is getting us into the shape of the goal He has for us, and yet over and over again we try to escape from the Sculptor's hand in an effort to batter ourselves into the shape of our own goal.

And he continues:

> The vision that God gives is not some unattainable castle in the sky, but a vision of what God wants you to be down here. Allow the Potter to put you on His wheel and whirl you around as He desires. Then as surely as God is God, and you are you, you will turn out as an exact likeness of the vision. Don't lose heart in the process. If you have ever had a vision from God, you may try as you will to be satisfied on a lower level, but God will never allow it.
>
> Isaiah 64:8 Yet, O LORD, you are our Father. We are the clay, you are the potter; we are all the work of your hand.
>
> Romans 9:21 Does not the potter have the right to make out of the same lump of clay some pottery for noble purposes and some for common use?

There are so many times that I resist being molded... It is the wrong time, I can do it better myself, that wouldn't work etc., but OH when I finally submit my "SELF," God once again proves that He knows what he is doing and when to do it. As I look back on this journey, I know ONLY GOD could/would handle a Battle such as this and be victorious. For without God I would have been running low on strength, courage, wisdom, patience or tenacity, really low.... not that I didn't sometimes but that must have been when I had let God slip out of focus. Thank you, Lord, for your very presence in my life.

Cathy

Praise God wherever you are and whatever situation He has allowed you to be in... His glory will shine through!

To: Cathy
From: Lisa F
Sent: Friday, July 7

Cathy,

I thought of you today when I received this... God Bless! God offers us "atomic bomb" power through Him, but often we go around leading only "firecracker" lives "[God]... is able to do immeasurably more than all we ask or imagine, according to His power that is at work in us." Ephesians 3:30

Lisa

[Friend from church]

To: Cathy
From: Beth
Sent: Friday, July 7

What an amazing, resilient, strong girl Molly is. Most of us would come home, curl up on the couch and feel sorry for ourselves. I am so in awe of her and in our God who is supplying her with this wonderful, powerful spirit.

Beth

To: Cathy
From: Kay L
Sent: Sunday, July 9

"Each day we learn from yesterday of God's great love and care;

and every burden we must face He'll surely help us bear." Quote by D. De Haan. It takes the storm to prove the real shelter.

Kay

To: Cathy
From: Jan
Sent: Sunday, July 9

Greetings from beautiful Vermont. I just want you to know I am thinking about you every day and Cath... What fabulous news I keep getting from you. I have to tell you again that I am so sorry all of you have had to have this ordeal, but I am learning so much from you and my love for you just grows. I hope Molly loves her job. cato

[This is one of my few friends who has been around long enough to call me by the same name as my mom did... Cath... A dear and wonderful faithful friend... She was one of those "safe" friends for Molly and hung out upstairs with her a couple of times and watched TV.]

[Week three of radiation treatment... at weeks' end she will have completed upper and lower field radiation leaving only the additional treatments to spleen and neck.]

To: Kitty
From: Cathy
Sent: Monday, July 10
Subject: Molly's fourth week of radiation

Good morning!
    We had a terrific lesson this week at church about what God is able to do. God has sure shown us his colors through this journey about his ability and yesterday a really good point was made.
    It is God who is able. Not us... It is through HIS STRENGTH,

HIS POWER, and HIS WISDOM through us that we get to the other side of whatever it is. For if we think WE CAN DO IT (overcome a sin, are successful at an endeavor, etc) then we get all pumped up in PRIDE. IF WE CAN'T DO IT, we get thrown into that pit of despair... BUT if we INVITE GOD to walk with us through life's changing seasons then IT IS HIS GLORY that shines through and we will be the ones who benefits.

I was thinking about walking with God. It is such an honor that we have that privilege. God, the creator of the universe and all things, is not only willing but available when we merely whisper his name. He comes along BESIDE us and empowers us through His Holy Spirit and truly satisfies our needs. Right then and there. Oh, your answer might not come immediately, but God's peace while you are waiting is overwhelming because you have transferred the control deal into His hands.

When we very first started this journey with Molly, I had a dream. Some of you have heard it but it is worth the repeat! It was a simple dream; I was standing alone, (not emotional) waiting. The backdrop was very tranquil (no bells and whistles). A figure appeared and handed me a rolled up piece of paper and simply stated: "This is the diagnosis." I took the piece of paper calmly and held it only for moments. Then on my right a bright and radiant form appeared (no face). He gently took the piece of paper and said "I'll handle this", and then He too was gone.

I have kept that image since the beginning. God is able and He has walked beside us with every stride. Even though I couldn't see him I knew He was there. By the notes He would put on your hearts to send, the sweet gestures, the perfect scripture verses, the sermons, the songs, the butterflies, the birds. God is with you too... just be expecting HIM to send YOU a little surprise to remind you of his presence.

These e-mails; I know many have enjoyed them and many have been so nice to come up and say sweet things, but I was reminded Sunday to give God all the credit for them, for it is God who has put these thoughts on my heart and it is God who has nudged me to write them down. This started quite simply and kept gaining momentum. It was His momentum; for this was a story of HIS glory.

As for you who are reading them; they are FOR YOU from God. Somehow, someway (God's way)! They are a reminder to you that no matter how strong your faith is, take a chance and be willing to let God change you. Be willing to let go of something you are holding tight to and let the God, who is able, take it upon His shoulders. This is not to be some preachy tactic but an honest implore for you to reach out into unfamiliar territory and give God a chance to fill you with HIS unimaginable love. For through it, you will be comforted and empowered and find a peace that truly passes all understanding.

One of the last thoughts in this sermon from church was LOVE AWAKENS LOVE. Let God love you, so you can love yourself and love others around you the way God has planned.

We had a Dr.'s appointment Friday. Molly is doing great! She turned 17 yesterday! Our last request to Dr. Paulino is that we NOT have to skip the week that was planned for radiation between the upper and lower fields. He said it depends on the counts on Monday and then we will make that decision. We go in for counts this morning at 9:30. Today will be the last of the 4 series treatments. We will only have 8 left after this one. There is a chance that we could be finished by next Thursday with all treatments (chemo and radiation). I am standing on GOOD COUNTS! Please stand with us through your prayers. God is ABLE, and my prayer is that he will enable her body as well!

Thank you always,
Cathy

Praise God wherever you are and whatever situation He has allowed you to be in... His glory will shine through!

From: Cathy
Sent: Monday, July 10
Subject: Good Counts

God did it again! We only have 8 more treatments after today. ALL treatments will be completed one week from Thursday. Her counts were GOOD... God is GREAT! And we are thrilled... Cathy

Praise God wherever you are or whatever situation He has allowed you to be in... His Glory will shine through.

Cathy

To: Cathy
From: Jan G
Sent: Monday, July 10

God is GOOD indeed! And to Him, Who is ABLE, all praise and glory!

Love and hugs,
Jan

To: Cathy
From: Pam
Sent: Monday, July 10

Thank you for your faithful updates about Molly. I thank God every day for the comfort and love that only He can give. Thinking of you each and every day with love and prayers.

Pam

To: Cathy
From: Kathe
Sent: July 10

Rejoicing with you all today! Thank you Lord!

love,
kathe

[This is another of my friends from church... she caught me in the hall one Sunday and said, "Cathy are you listening, you really need to compile these and publish these . . ." It is funny but that was the clear moment that I realized that this might be what God has planned to do with this story.]

To: Cathy
From: Blake
Sent: Monday, July 10

That's Awesome! Good for Molly!

Blake

[My son in law married to Jamie Ann]

To: Cathy
From: Paula
Sent: Monday, July 10

You have always known, but realize now what a gift each day is and how precious friends and family really, really are.

May God continue to shine His Glory on you, Molly, Mel and the rest of your family. And what a glorious time you will have to rejoice on the trip to California!!!

Your family has been an inspiration to all of us.

Love and Thanks,
Paula

[This is my church friend who has a dry dry sense of wonderful humor. She once told me that she washed her dishes to please the Lord... I still remember where she was sitting when she said it... I though it so odd, and that she surely was kidding... that was 25 years ago and finally years later I understood what she meant.... do everything unto the Lord... and never will you be disappointed by expectations. For his blessings are abundant... and His love enfolds me... even when I am doing menial everyday tasks]

To: Cathy
From: Anita
Sent: Monday, July 10

Once again, thank you for including me on the list and for keeping me informed. Molly and all of you all are never far from my thoughts and hope that this will all be behind you very soon. I have never gotten away from September being the real beginning of the New Year. I hope that September finds you healthy, happy and ready for a new school year.

Nita

[Sweet friend and mom of 2 daughters]

To: Cathy
From: Jan G
Sent: Tuesday, July 11

"How privileged I am to be indwelt by your glorious presence (by the whole Trinity: Father, Son and Holy Spirit!) so I can display your excellence to those around me." You reflect the very essence of this. As you walk in the blessed assurance and grace and mercy of our Abba Father, you are a walking demonstration to each of us that Satan is a defeated foe. Through the transparency of your hearts you have allowed us to witness what it is to live as victors NOT as victims! It is impossible for you to comprehend the impact you have on each of us. Your steadfast faith and courage have inspired, uplifted and renewed all who have had the honor to come along side you and stand in the gap. Thank you for allowing us to share in God's amazing grace as we lift you up and witness the miraculous ways He works through every detail of every circumstance.

Love,
Jan

To: Cathy
From: Terri S
Sent: Tuesday, July 11

Dear Cathy, thank you so much for taking the time to write these encouraging words to us. We know your heart and know that you always give God the glory. You truly encourage me. I take your words, close my eyes and think about my situations and apply the instruction or sweet thoughts or images you write. You are helping me in a personal way. I do appreciate the help. I hope this morning went well for Molly. Her struggle is helping many people and bringing us closer to Him. I am sending much love and prayer your way…

Terri

To: Cathy
From: Lou Ann
Sent: Tuesday, July 11

Dear Molly and Cathy:
 So happy to hear about the great counts and Molly's new job! A friend sent me this prayer and I thought of you. Lou Ann
 P.S. A prayer from Mother Theresa: "Today may there be peace within. May you trust God that you are exactly where you are meant to be. May you not forget the infinite possibilities that are born of faith. May you use those gifts that you have received, and pass on the love that has been given to you. May you be content knowing you are a child of God. Let his presence settle into your bones, and

allow your soul the freedom to sing, dance, praise and love. It is there for each and every one of us."

To: Cathy
From: Lynn R
Sent: Tuesday, July 11

Thank you for the update! I cannot wait to read the other emails. I have not wanted to bother you, but you are constantly in my thoughts and prayers. I am in awe of your strength and so blessed to call you "friend."

Lynn

[Just a note: Lynn and her husband John were also at the wedding that you read about in the beginning of this book. We had been at the reception just long enough to hug the bride and groom, visit with a few friends, and speak to the T's... but it was time to head out, our hearts were heavy and we just needed a peaceful quiet spot to regain our thoughts. Knowing the jolts of the week, Lynn and John invited us to come to their house for a glass of wine. The four of us sat outside on their stone deck as a blazing fire in the outdoor fireplace warmed our hearts and settled our souls. Mel and I talked through some of the fears and concerns that were clamoring in our minds and we needed that! I don't think they even knew how much we truly appreciated their support and that kind gesture. Oh but we did!]

To: Cathy
From: Jill
Sent: Tuesday, July 11

Precious Cathy,

I have a scripture that I want you to read that is Molly's song as well as the Psalmist's. (Psalms 118: 1, 14–17, 21, 29) I hope all went well today.

I love you,
Jill

To: Kitty
From: Cathy
Date: Wednesday, July 12
Subject: Appreciate EACH Birthday

We have five family birthdays this month, all exactly one week apart. Wouldn't you know that each would be on a Sunday this year? First Molly, then Tom, then Mel and then Jamie Ann and Blake (they have exactly the same birthday). Each celebration will be different according to the one to whom we are celebrating. They have different likes and different needs. Each one of them is loved so greatly, and it is THEIR life we are celebrating. Molly's birthday this year brought light to me of a whole new perspective of appreciation for each BIRTHDAY. There is a precious spot that each child holds that no one can replace.

So it is with God I think... He celebrates with joy each life he has created. He molds each of us according to our different bents, using ways and adversities specifically suited to strengthen characteristics he intends to use for his glory here on earth.

Tom, (our only son... and one terrific one might I add) and I had this big discussion on character last week. We talk a lot and have some pretty wonderful discussions. I said that I thought basic character stands and reoccurs. He said, "Mom, look at the people in the bible. Look at Moses. He said 'No, I can't lead your people.' Paul, 'I detest Jesus Christ.' Jonah, 'I don't want to go and deliver your message.' But they all were changed by God. He is right; character is able to be changed. Because when you study those characters and so many others in the bible God has made drastic changes in their character, beliefs and perspectives."

Basic character can be molded and matured and actually changed. For it is by God's AUTHORITY that he incurs change. He makes changes in us internally to reflect HIS glory externally. Jesus Christ celebrates your life. I suspect that there is a bunch inside of you and me that has not yet been handed over to him to govern and have authority over. Each of us is uniquely made with quirks, habits, gifts, looks, selfish ways, etc., but we are all created by the same God of Glory for the same intention: TO GLORIFY HIM, in All that we do. Overwhelming thought for me! I glorify him some of the time, but oh I can sure get on my high horse and ride with MY AUTHORITY.

God has proclaimed His Authority over and over to me and ON me, especially during this journey. It has been so clear. Just remember that God celebrates His creation of you. You are so special and there is no one on this earth that can take your place. Think about giving him the Authority to make some changes. It is a little uncomfortable to let someone else do the leading of YOUR life but I speak from the fires that we have walked through these past few months. We have not only been protected from scorch but we have been blessed by HIS GLORY.

Prayer Request:
Lower Field is tougher than we thought. Please pray for a strong and tolerant stomach
Praise that we can see the end... only 7 more treatments!

Cathy

Praise God wherever you are and whatever situation He has allowed you to be in... His glory will shine through!

To: Cathy
From: Ruth Ann
Sent: Wednesday, July 12

Amen, in ALL things He is sufficient and He is victorious! Praise Him for the wonder He is working in and through Molly and late and very happy birthday! How we will celebrate your life and His life in you.

Love,
Ruth Ann

[This precious lady is another of my mentors. Her wisdom and her tenacity are ever present but it is her faithfulness and obedience to God that is glaring to me as an example of how to live.]

To: Cathy
From: Gina
Sent: Wednesday, July 12

Sometimes I wonder why God allows struggle in our lives... and then I realize that He is using Cathy to further His Kingdom... her emails are reaching Norway... I only wonder where they travel after Europe... maybe even some of the military camps of the Middle East.... and some missionary villages in Africa or educational dorms in China... to God be the Glory...

love,
gina

[Always an encourager]

To: Kitty
From: Cathy
Sent: Thursday, July 13
Subject: PLEASE.... Thank Kitty

Dear friends—please join me in thanking Kitty for the time she has spent editing, sending, responding, gathering comments and truly being one of God's messengers. She is a dear friend and picked up a ball that I had no idea was even rolling and threw it out among you. She allowed me the privilege of sharing my thoughts, updates and prayer requests as she accepted the role of our catalyst and dear friend. There are no words of appreciation that would be adequate, so I pray that she will know in her heart how deeply appreciative we are for her and to her.

Kitty, I love you to pieces and finally have figured out how to send these e-mails. You have been the most precious friend through all of this—you have held us up at times when not even you knew it—you have been diligent, loyal, dependable, insightful and a true messenger. Thank you for your tenacity. We are closing in to the end and it is time for me to take responsibility of a chore that you have so unselfishly tackled. I suspect that there will be only a few e-mails left to this group list... so I will send them from here. You have been and are such an inspiration to me and I ask God to BLESS you greatly for holding our hand in such a gentle way as we have waded through this river.

May you be constantly in the protection of our Almighty God and may your life continue to radiate His presence which dwells within you,

I Love you,
Cathy

Praise God wherever you are, or whatever situation He has allowed you to be in... His Glory will shine through.

To: Cathy
From: Susan K
Sent: Thursday, July 13
Subject: Birthday E-mail

I hate to keep harping on this, but I think you have missed your calling. You are the most beautiful writer or rather you put things so beautifully into words. Your email yesterday about the birthdays was so touching. I think I will always look at birthdays differently. Throughout all of this you have been so sweet to take the time to let us all know your personal journey. You have truly been a messenger of God. You and Molly have touched so many people. I have a few people that don't even know you and ask me to send your emails. I will miss your emails; they have been so uplifting and filled with so much love and faith. I will continue to pray for precious Molly. I am just so happy that things have gone so well. I know she is excited about her new job too. I hope these last seven treatments just fly by and that she feels healthy and strong when they are through. Thank you, thank you, thank you and to Kitty for all of her hard work. She is so wonderful. God Bless you all!

Love,
Susan

[There were many e-mails that were sent in reply to my e-mail thanking Kitty for her dedication: These two seem to sum up the praise of many!]

To: Cathy for Kitty
From: Terri S
Sent: Thursday, July 13

Dearest Kitty, you truly are God's instrument. What is that verse about when one falls down your friend will hold you up? That is you! I spoke to you early in the summer about printing out all of these instructional emails for me to read and study. Thank you for your unselfish devotion to Cathy.

Love,
Terri

To: Cathy for Kitty
From: Kay L
Sent: Thursday, July 13
Wisdom You are seeing Ecclesiastes 4:7–12 with 12 being the cord of 3 lived out. The living version is so sweet too. And also the verse (cannot remember the address) of standing in the gap with prayer for a friend. Have a blessed day as you get to the end of this week.

Love,
K

[We are there... home stretch, Monday, Tuesday, Wednesday and

Thursday... Then she is through with ALL of her treatments... PRAISE GOD... our Almighty Friend and Deliverer.

From: Cathy
Sent: Monday, July 17
Subject: Wooden Angel

A funny guy, a senior saint at our church named Bud sent Molly a little wooden angel with metal wings kneeling in prayer when we first began this journey. I put it on the sofa table in the den and pass it and see it probably 10 times a day. Yesterday I was thanking him for it and realized that little angel has stayed right in her place (like she could walk or something).

It reminded me that God too has been right there in his spot the whole time too. He DID move. He was in Molly's room when she was by herself, He was in the treatment room when she was having radiation, He was with me during quiet times, and He was with Mel while He was making hard decisions. Though He was not so tangible as that little angel, He made Himself quite visible through friends, and hospital staff, and birds, thoughts on my heart, time lines, willingness for Dr.'s to try new protocols and ways to do things, regenerating blood cells to just the right counts, he was there... in every step and every move.

God's promise to be with us forever is HIS WORD and he stands by it at every interval, over and over again—Dueteronomy 26:8 "The LORD himself goes before you and will be with you; he will never leave you nor forsake you. Do not be afraid; do not be discouraged." Do we recognize Him when He takes on such different roles? Or do we expect Him in just one or two ways and limit our minds to comprehend how vast His presence is and how mighty He is. We serve a God who knows US, each one of us. He knows how we are wired. He knows our needs and questions and doubts and fears and inadequacies and our sins, and man do we all have some. He stands right there to CONQUER our stuff through His Son and His Holy Spirit who dwells inside of us.

Sometimes I think I can pull it off myself but one of the things I have been forced to learn through this journey is this: It is too much trouble to try to do this myself. First of all, the load is way too heavy. And second, I don't know the road or the directions or even the next destination. I have found that on this journey, one task sets you up to handle the next one. So if God knows the road, knows the directions and knows the destination, what am I thinking if I don't ask for him to come along? Guess I'm not!

We are winding down on these e-mails. I hope that you will consider some of the lessons that God has given me to share. If by chance you aren't practicing any of them, just try to look at things through different lens, namely God's. It is funny how clear things become sometimes when you change the way you look at them.

Specific Prayers:
This radiation is messing with her stomach big time—only 3 more days—just pray for her to have a settled mind, spirit and body We will follow up with a Dr.'s appointment back at Texas Children's on Wednesday, July 26. She will have her PICC line removed. Please pray for smooth sailing on that. Praise to God for the details he has continued to work out and work through during this process.

Thank you,
Cathy

Praise God wherever you are and whatever situation He has allowed you to be in...His glory will shine through!

To: Cathy
From: Sandy
Sent: Monday, July 17

I am so glad that you are nearing the end of your journey. Seeing the wondrous ways that God has worked out all the details for you is so encouraging...because it's been such an inspiration to know that He is actually doing the same in all of our lives! You have been a shining example to all. God's love and light have definitely shown through you and Molly. Love, Sandy P.S. A big thank you also goes to Kitty for sharing with us!

Sandy

[Gina hosts a bible study in her home each year when we take a summer break... Meg R. teaches and this is where I met Sandy.]

To: Cathy
From: Helene
Sent: Monday, July 17

I can't believe this horrible ordeal is nearly over. My heart feels so light just thinking about it. How faithful our God is! You have been such a living testament to not only His healing powers, His power to do absolutely anything, but also to His complete faithfulness and His love for us. You and your entire family have almost crossed out of the Valley of the Shadow of Death; you can see and feel and smell the other side... what joy!

Helene

To: Cathy
From: Kay S
Sent: Monday, July 17

Cathy, this has been a journey that I would have NEVER wanted for any of you, but you are now at the end and the witness that each of you has been is without words to describe. I went to "L" yesterday to spend the night with Mom and we talked about you and Molly so much. She has been praying for your sweet girl faithfully (like so many others) and while I was driving home today, I just had the most sobering thought—you didn't have your mom to lean on during this time. Cathy, I am so sorry for that but I know Our Heavenly Father meets every need we have. I love you my friend and cannot wait to just praise God when this is all behind you and sweet

Molly is "kicking up her heels" because she has forgotten what it feels like to "feel good."

Sending you hugs,
kay

[My friend of encouragement]

To: Cathy
From: Bonnie C
Sent: Monday, July 17

Dearest Cathy:
    I have been praying for you. Even thought I have been quiet, I have been there in thought everyday, right beside you. First thing I would do each morning is read Kitty's devotional, and you or your friends' reports. There are times when I felt like I could just reach out and hug you and Molly and your family at any moment. Thank you for including me on your journeys this past year. Hope to see you soon.

Infinity,
Bonnie

[This is my childhood partner in crime who now lives in College Station…she was and still is my dear friend. When we were children, we would always end our conversations with "infinity"… because we didn't want our friendship to ever end and it never did…And it never will!]

To: Cathy
From: Mary Leslie
Sent: Monday, July 17

Cathy,
    You have truly made me look at the simple ways God connects

us to Him... your insight and sensitivity to His presence brings us to not only his Word, but His presence in our everyday life experiences. My life has slowed down with Craig's* illness and I am beginning to be more sensitive to the journey everyday... to people, to the beauty in nature and to new relationships.... some are very brief, but they all touch me in some way. Thank you Lord for challenges in life that allow me to see your presence in new each day. My prayers continue every day for precious Molly and all of you.

Our prayers continue everyday for them!

Mary Leslie

[Note: Craig is Mary Leslie's husband who has been fighting an Auto Immune disease called Polymyositis with associated interstitial lung disease. It affects the muscles in his body. They have been struggling with this disease for a year now and are still unable to find a suitable cure.]

To: Molly's Prayer Warriors
From: Cathy
Sent: Tuesday, July 18, 2006
Subject: Chewing the Worry

Bentley, Molly's adolescent lab, (6 months 50 lbs—yellow lab), lost her good dog focus the other day and decided to take one of those red styrofoam swimming noodles and chew it to pieces (literally)— This didn't bother me much but had Mel seen it, being the orderly guy he is, he wouldn't have taken to kindly to it. So I picked up the pieces, all 100 of them or so and thought: this is what I do to God. I take my focus off of doing what is right and good and chew into pieces a worry or situation until I have pretty much covered the entire thought and just made a terrible mess of my emotions.
If I just could have caught Bentley early. We could have avoided the clean up! And if I just could stop the thoughts early, I could avoid the wear and tear of FRET.

So how do I stop them early? SUBSTITUTE one thought for another! Your mind can only have one basic thought at a time, so instead of giving into one that makes you crazy with worry or unease, think about GOD and His things on this Earth that are excellent and things in your life that are blessings.

> Phillipians 4:8 Finally, brothers, whatever is true, whatever is noble, whatever is right, whatever is pure, whatever is lovely, whatever is admirable—if anything is excellent or praiseworthy—think about such things.

It truly works! It takes a little time to make a habit out of it, but if you keep training your mind you will soon be convinced that this is an easier way to live. So many of the things we worry about never even happen, and so many of the circumstances are things we really have no control over... So why not just go on and LET GOD HANDLE THEM.

Over these last few months I have chewed and chewed some thoughts into little bitty pieces. Finally I have had to give it up and think of the things of excellence and the many blessings we have been given. God gladly takes the wheel of our boat, but He isn't going to fight for it. He wants you to ask for help and He always is just a blink away!

Cathy

Praise God where ever you are and whatever situation He has allowed you to be in... His glory will shine through!

To: Cathy
From: Jan G
Sent: Tuesday, July 18
Subject: Faith and Grace

I awoke this morning at 5:30 with this thought going through my head—move over Batman and Robin, here come Faith and Grace! It was crystal clear to me that the two of you represent Faith and Grace. Cathy, your faithfulness in sharing your heart thoughts with us and Kitty your grace in forwarding Cathy's "journal" and the comments of so many prayer warriors have impacted lives across our country and beyond! I am reminded of what we do on Christmas

Eve in church... In complete darkness, we all hold candles and with only one flame to begin, within minutes the entire sanctuary is filled with light. You have filled our lives with the light of the world!

You have shown us the compassionate, unwavering commitment our Lord and Savior desires for each of us if we just let go and "let God." With a grateful heart, I thank you for your obedience to Him and for showering your faith and grace on me. I love you and always hold you close to my heart.

Jan

To: Cathy
From: Ruth Ann
Sent: Tuesday, July 18

Amen to His knowing all and being able to guide us and take the BEST care of us! Our love and prayers as you COMPLETE these treatments!

RuthAnn

To: Cathy (Mom)
From: Jennifer
Sent: Tuesday, July 18

I loved this email. Maybe the best of all! I could retell this lesson using Kirby. She'll tear up any number of things; her puppy pads, any box or cardboard she can get a hold of, Jon's new toothbrush from the dentist, my Gerber daisies (she actually gets up on the kitchen table to "pick" flowers and shred them on the floor).

But I especially loved your message. It resonates well with me. That's how I do it. This is how I get through crumby work days and family frustrations. I just choose to substitute my thoughts with something else. It works really well, for a while. The problem with me is that I do it myself. I don't substitute with God. I think about productive things; which are better than the alternative, but not enough to sustain me. That's when I crater. I've learned this about myself. I can keep it up for long time, but when I fall, I fall hard because I have been depending on myself instead of on God.

For me the hardest part is time. I know what to do. Better yet, I know what God can do. But I don't make time to listen to Him. Devotionals are a good way to start the day. They get you thinking about God early in the day. They set your mind on the right things. But to truly learn to depend on Him, you have to do more than read about him. You have to trust Him. You have to listen to Him. You have to allow Him to talk to you and guild your steps.

As I get older, I hope that I can learn from your example and listen to God talk. Most people don't hear Him like you do. You are an inspiration. Your notes have been personal, heartfelt and honest. They have glorified God. And I don't think I have told you how much I have enjoyed them. Thank you mom!

Love,
Jennifer

[From my daughter... this is so precious for a mom to hear]

To: Cathy
From: Ann W
Sent: Tuesday, July 18

I just wish I had been hearing your emails all along. What an impact, as you say when you have lived it and seen it. I am saving these to share at the right time. I remember when I was doing Child Advocates. After several years, I really felt like it was time to leave (I didn't know God was behind those kind of things at the time.) I felt so guilty I felt that way. Finally I decided I just had to quit and it took several months to wind what I was doing down. During that time, Janie asked me to teach the night class. I could never have done both. To me, it was a good lesson that there are many good things we can do for God, but what He wants is for us to just be obedient to His leadings, even if our brains try to tell us no. Only He knows the perfect path He has planned for us. I'm so glad God put you on my heart permanently many years ago. Go girl! We'll keep up from time to time and will have eternity to have wonderful talks.

Love you.
Ann

[This is my tennis friend from way back...a seasoned bible study teacher and a heart that craves the Lord]

To: Cathy
From: Allison
Sent: Tuesday, July 18

Thank you, Cathy, for that reminder that God does not want us to fret, but to focus on Him. Your email came at a perfect time for me!

love,
allison

To: Molly's Prayer Warriors
From: Cathy
Sent: Wednesday, July 19
Subject: God Stayed With Us

Yesterday morning Molly and I were riding to Methodist and I told Molly what an honor it has been to walk beside her as she weathered this storm. I told her of the patience, the courage, perseverance, poise and beauty I had witnessed as she tackled whatever was thrown her way, and that I just loved her to pieces. (Can't you see the "where is this going" sign flashing in her mind... and she's stuck)I now know her, can tell you her habits, what bugs her, can read her face and she knows all that about me. I said: "Molly, I am really proud of you!" She replied, "Thanks for staying with me, Mom."

We have spent "every single day... and evening at some point together"... I know her and she knows me. Guess now you can see where I am going with this. When you spend a bunch of time over and over with someone, you begin to know their quirks, their habits, what makes them happy and what sends them up a wall. You know when they are up or down or in the middle and what their likes and dislikes are... you just know them.

God so wants us to KNOW HIM... but we can only know Him by being with Him; "everyday... and evening at some point." Molly has been dependent on Mel and I. She has weathered this storm with God's hand upon her and with your many prayers but she has needed support mentally, physically and spiritually as well and so do we!

> You want someone to love you to pieces—God Does
> You want someone to be there when the storms come crashing through—God Is
> You want someone to forget/forgive the stupid mean things you have done—God Has
> You want someone to go before you and lead your way—God Will
> You want someone who keeps promises, answers calls, returns calls, is never in a hurry, understands your heartache, appreciates your gifts, knows your disappointments, overcomes sorrow, bestows grace, smiles with favor, transmits wisdom, shares joy and never quits—GOD is the one—the one and only and He is just a whisper away.

We have all had to be dependent on God, each one of us in our family. For this was a family trip! Complete with blow outs, pit stops, snacks, and song. We invited God to drive, and He has driven toward each horizon, which was new to us but old hat for Him, with awesome candor. We are forever grateful that GOD STAYED WITH US but especially that He has held Molly so closely and gently in His arms.

With great love and appreciation to God and to
you dear prayer warriors,
Cathy

Praise God wherever you are and whatever situation He has allowed you to be in... His glory will shine through!

To: Cathy
From: Mel [my husband]
Sent: Wednesday, July 19

Thank you for your wisdom of today. I find the same, for as I discuss God on Wednesday mornings before work, it is reflected in my attitude toward work and how I respond to daily challenges. So if we develop a daily relationship with God, our lives and impact on others will be improved, no matter what the winds might blow our way... I love you and thank you for being Molly's rock throughout this ordeal...

Just a note: Mel has been the rock for all of us! He was there at most all of Molly's chemo appointments, and Dr's appointments. He remained steady when my emotions seemed to be in dismay. He was the first to say "What can I do" and always showed loving concern and compassion for what his precious Molly was going through. He was our Rock on Earth, I was only the pebble... for I could often times get shoved around by the current. His feet were planted... and he was clearly being guided by the Lord. I am thankful that God gave me a man of integrity, steadfastness, loyalty, love and responsibility to be my husband and the dad of our children. For all of us are proud to be one of His Jodeit's! God has blessed us greatly through the love and leadership of this precious man. He is a blessing to us all and we thank him... I do especially!

Mel

To: Cathy
From: Susan I
Sent: Wednesday, July 19

Thank you Cathy, for the witness to God's faithfulness you've been for me. As we have been going through our own trials, your insights and testimony to God's goodness in the midst of suffering has buoyed me up. I praise God with you for bringing Molly and your family through this fire, coming out as gold.

Love,
Susan

To: Cathy
From: JoAnn
Sent: Wednesday, July 19

Hi Cathy.

You know that that Philippians verse is ONE OF MY MOST FAVORITES! Thanks for the great e-mail and analogy with Bentley; a great visual and I love visuals and God's Word together. The Lord is really using you and your "examples" to give all of us who are blessed to read your e-mails and pray for you a practical view of His Word in our life. I'm thinking and praying for you all on your "home stretch."....jojo "REJOICE IN HOPE, ENDURE IN AFFLICTION, PERSEVERE IN PRAYER" Romans 12:12

JoAnn

To: Molly's Prayer Warriors
From: Cathy
Sent: Thursday, July 20
Subject: Last Day Molly

Today is the last day of treatments for Molly—this journey is coming to an end...

When something is over, don't you sometimes find yourself thinking about when it began...It is kind of like a trip except this one was quite last minute. You pack fast, move fast and then you're going. While you're on your way you think about what is going to happen when you get there. You try to think one step ahead but if the territory is unfamiliar you really have no base for thought, and the anxiousness starts to bubble. Think about the last time you had to do something that was way out of your comfort zone. You really do move at a step by step pace evaluating and calculating road maps.

"Road map" was a familiar phrase used these past few months. This was the route used to accomplish the goal of annihilating the cancer in Molly's body. It didn't matter how much faith we had. This shook our world. Maybe it did matter, but I didn't have enough to not be ruffled.

Mel and I knew that we were accountable for making good decisions for Molly and HER TRUST IN US was without question. We tackled the usual traveling dilemmas; the arrival, the baggage, the vehicle for transportation, the traffic, etc. But we traveled without delay or detour. I asked God at the beginning to let us get through this process without interruption. We not only had no interruptions, we were early! Looking back is a good thing. You can reflect on specific highlights that you were often going too fast to notice. We often times tend to become distracted with something more essential at that moment to take notice of the blessings at hand. I know that as surely as Molly TRUSTED US—WE WERE TRUSTING GOD. We were not versed in this arena.

I wish I could say that I didn't question the next step or ask, "God, are you sure you are with us here?"... because I did. God just stayed His steady self, and He tried to steady me. IT IS TRUE... when you find yourself wavering if you focus on God who is so rock solid, it gives you a comfort and confidence to hold your head up high and KNOW without any doubt that this too will pass! The bottom line is: God's Glory will shine triumphantly.

This trip is almost over, at least the treatment part. How many times have you heard it said that you wouldn't wish this trial on anyone but the blessings received from it are without measure? We are all changed. That is what traveling does to you. It gives you a different perspective because you have been on foreign unfamiliar soil. Your comfort zone has been challenged. When all is said and done, I have said that I wish that I could have been the one who had to carry this burden. After seeing how Molly handled it, I discovered that it was me that needed to learn lessons that God could only teach me through Molly. Trusting God with Molly was vastly different than trusting God with me...children are such elusive treasures.

She is one of mine...But even more so she is one of God's.—And there is no trace of elusiveness to God; he knows her every moment.

> Psalm 114 He has caused his wonders to be remembered;
> the LORD is gracious and compassionate.

Cathy

Praise God wherever you are and whatever situation He has allowed you to be in...His glory will shine through!

To: Cathy
From: Mary Leslie
Sent: Thursday, July 20

Lots of praises today for a journey you allowed us to see through email pictures we hold in our hearts and minds. I know Molly and each of you has a peace that merits some "let down time" and I hope that you experience some rest now...we love you ...

Mary Leslie

[They are fighting their own battles with her husband Craig's disease...but ML is always thinking of others]

It is Finished

IT IS OVER... Molly is my forever hero... she has fought a difficult journey with beauty, poise, tenacity, patience, courage, endurance, charm and honor. I salute her courage, we all do... for she has been an example of the mighty strength of prayer and a witness to the mighty hand of God that has been upon her!

To: Molly's Prayer Warriors
From: Cathy
Sent: Thursday, July 20
Subject: It Is Finished...

IT IS FINISHED... In the Methodist Radiation Oncology Lobby there is a Brass Captain's Bell mounted on the wall and there is a sign that reads:

> Ring this bell
> 3 times well
> a toll to dearly say-
>
> My treatments done
> This course is run
> and I am on my way!
>
> J.L. Kennington 11/00

You see this sign at first glance when you enter the lobby area for your first consultation. Through the process of how ever many weeks, you have a chance to see folks RING THAT BELL. You are so glad for them and think one day it will be our turn. You know it's not really the bell that you are looking forward to it is what the bell represents. We got to the hospital about 10:30, usual time, but today was different—we had made cookies for the parking guys, had surprises for the radiation staff and cookies for Dr. Paulino.

Tom, Mel, Jennifer, Jamie and her baby were all there to witness the ringing of the bell. Molly didn't know they were coming and Tom arrived first and Molly was so appreciative to him for being there. He said with that great big smile of his, "I heard you get to 'Ring the Bell' today and I wanted to be here to see it!" Then came Jamie then Jennifer and Mel. Yeah, we were all there. Molly was glad they were there. This time it wasn't about attention but of victory. They all had helped her get through this ordeal, each offered a different approach. The staff came out to watch and she rang the bell with pride. This brought a little bit of closure to what had been a hard fought battle for Molly and all of us. We celebrate this victory with God and our dear friends who have stood steady beside us as we tackled this challenge.

Think about what you are dealing with… and the battle you are fighting! When God allows a battle to come your way, put on your armor and BE BRAVE in the Lord.

> The Armor of God—Ephesians 6
>
> Finally, be strong in the Lord and in his mighty power. Put on the full armor of God so that you can take your stand against the devil's schemes.
> For our struggle is not against flesh and blood, but against the rulers, against the authorities, against the powers of this dark world and against the spiritual forces of evil in the heavenly realms.
> Therefore put on the full armor of God, so that when the day of evil comes, you may be able to stand your ground, and after you have done everything, to stand. Stand firm then, with the belt of truth buckled around your waist, with the breastplate of righteousness in place,

and with your feet fitted with the readiness that comes
from the gospel of peace.
In addition to all this, take up the shield of faith, with
which you can extinguish all the flaming arrows of the
evil one.
Take the helmet of salvation and the sword of the Spirit,
which is the word of God.
And pray in the Spirit on all occasions with all kinds
of prayers and requests. With this in mind, be alert and
always keep on praying for all the saints.

Make a conscious effort to resort to God's ways and not your own. One day you too will get to ring your bell and those who you have trusted to help pray you through will too be standing with you to celebrate.

Molly has requested "Home made Dressing" for dinner so we have turned tonight's dinner into a THANKSGIVING dinner—with turkey from Goode Co, home made dressing... and some extras. Our whole family will all be gathered to Praise God and Thank Him for the way He has guided, lifted, pushed, and pulled Molly and all of us through this maze called cancer.

It is with deepest appreciation to all of you from the whole Jodeit Family for your support through your prayers and encouragement. God has blessed us with treasured friends and we are forever grateful to each of you.

May God bless you with his mighty hand upon you,
May He show you the way when times are dark,
May His love embrace you when loneliness grips you,
May His wisdom fall upon you in time of need
May His peace penetrate down deep in your soul,
May His joy overflow as you allow Him to be your friend.
and...
May His smile be upon you for what you have done on our behalf.

Lord let us take this story, and the lessons you have taught us through it and pass it on so that others will see your Glory.

Blessings abound and thanks be to God for giving us this Bell Ringing Day,

Love,
Cathy

Praise God wherever you are and whatever situation He has allowed you to be in... His glory will shine through!

To: Cathy
From: Debbie E
Sent: Thursday, July 20

Cathy,

Don't be surprised if you have an unexpected wave of emotions in the next week (or month) or two. After you have geared up for a fight like this, and stayed strong, after it's over, you get to let go. It caught me totally by surprise, and it may not happen to you, but if it does, just know that it's normal and it passes fairly quickly. It's relief and emotional release combined with letting go. I'm good in a crisis, and I fall apart later—so it may just be me—but just wanted to share in case you go through it, too.

Cancer changes your perspective on things forever, and in a good way. You also meet some very wonderful medical personnel along the way, don't you? Congratulations to all of you on getting to this point in your journey.

Lots of Love,
Deb

[Debbie is a friend from Junior High School, who also has had cancer and is now in remission... when she said cancer changes your perspective forever... nothing could be truer!]

To: Cathy
From: Cynthia
Sent: Thursday, July 20

Oh, my... I'm just crying with joy! Praise God and yea Molly! I, too, would have loved to have been there to hear the crisp, strong ring of the bell. I will be joining with you in Thanksgiving over this milestone in all of your lives. Hope that the rest of her summer... and yours will be the best ever.

I love you all,
C

[She was joining us with Thanksgiving as so many were]

To: Cathy
From: Wanda
Sent: Thursday, July 20

Dearest Cathy and Molly,
 Reminds me of "It's a Wonderful Life" when the little bell rings and Jimmy Stewart says, "Every time a bell rings, an angel gets his wings." Molly has received her wings, and I pray she will soar to heights that she never could have realized had she not fought through this struggle and been lifted by the diligent prayers of those who have so lovingly lifted her every day before the throne of our Lord and Savior. May life be sweeter, those you love be dearer, and the little joys God sends never again be overlooked.

Love,
Wanda

[My church friend... and our Pastor's right hand administrator]

To: Cathy
From: Kathy O
Sent: Thursday, July 20

Praises, praises... God's glory is shining through! I am so happy for Molly and your entire family that this is over! It has been a privilege to be a part of this journey. Many thanks!

Kathy

To: Cathy
From: Debbie K
Sent: Thursday, July 20

You have truly been a blessing to me with these word-picture e-mails describing the journey your family has had with God these past months! Thank you for your words, and for your honesty. You have enabled all those who love the Jodeit's to pray specifically for what you need, and at the same time, you have taught invaluable life lessons and God lessons to each of us. I will continue to pray for all of you, and of course for Molly.

　　Thank you for your friendship and for trusting me with your prayer requests, but also, thank you for these devotionals through which I grow closer to understanding what God offers me.

In love and prayer,
Debbie

Psalm 111:4 He has caused his wonders to be remembered; the LORD is gracious and compassionate.

To: Cathy
From: Georgiana
Sent: Thursday, July 20

Dear Cathy,

I have been thinking of you all day today. Thank God this is all over! Molly must be so relieved to be finished. You have handled this with such courage and have been such and example to me and everyone else following your journey. Call me if you want to go for a walk some morning. I love you.

Georgiana

To: Cathy
From: Helene
Sent: Thursday, July 20

This is a very special day for your family, for Molly and for God... a day of relief, introspection and celebration. I know God is so happy and proud. You are His people and you have come through the desert, stronger in faith and overflowing with praise. You are an inspiration and a blessing to me.

Love,
Helene

To: Cathy
From: Nancy
Sent: Thursday, July 20

Cathy, the Lord is good, and has certainly been a steadfast "travel agent" during this most harrowing of journeys - praise the Lord for raising Molly safely to this point—you all remain in our prayers—love,

Nancy

[The word raising got my attention... you know what I mean?]

To: Cathy
From: Kathy B
Sent: Wednesday, July 20

I am SO very happy that Molly is finished with her treatment; she has been a hero to everyone who has gone along on your journey. Speaking from experience I know how scary cancer can be—but, you have all faced it with such courage and grace that it has been an inspiration to us all. I will pray for continued strength and peace for all of you!

Hugs,
Kathy

[A friend and cancer survivor who has first hand knowledge of the kind of courage and grace that God supplies]

To: Cathy
From: Jill
Sent: Thursday, July 20

Cathy,

I am sure that this is undoubtedly the most thankful Thanksgiving that the Jodeit family has ever had together! Praise God!

Jill

To: Cathy
From: Mel
Sent: Thursday, July 20

Excellent message... Such wisdom... Now I understand why you beat me at gin last night... It was by the grace of God... HA!
    Note here: We often times play gin rummy in the evenings... I used to think I was good but my track record of losing so many

consecutive games in a row has caused me to reevaluate. He is the champ... no doubt, in card playing as well as in my life.

Mel

To: Cathy
From: Rob
Sent: Thursday, July 20

"Next thing you know it will all be over"—-see ya'—your pal

[This is a friend who I have worked for and with for six or so years. He was and is a great cheerleader for many who have needed encouragement. God knew I would need his one liners and his positive outlook... and he always has a smile to share. He told me at the beginning of this journey to just take one day at a time and one day I will look at it and it will be all over. He was right... I remembered his words often. He is a wonderful friend and I thank him!]

To: Cathy
From: Tom S (my brother)
Sent: Thursday, July 20

I am so happy!!! Molly is a real trooper and so are all her family members........Congrats!!!!!!!!

Tom

To: Cathy
From: Georgiana
Sent: Thursday, July 20

Dear Cathy,
 I have been thinking of you all day today. Thank God this is all over! Molly must be so relieved to be finished. You have handled

this with such courage and have been such an example to me and everyone else following your journey. Call me if you want to go for a walk some morning. I love you.

Georgiana

To: Cathy
From: Lisa C
Sent: Thursday, July 20

Praise the Lord! We are so happy fro Molly that she is finished! What a trying time she has had. We are thankful she is done! Have a wonderful celebration with your family, you all deserve it! Cathy Thank you so much for all of your wonderful uplifting scriptures! You are great; I don't know what I am going to do without having new ones to read. If you ever want to continue them, please send them my way... all of the prayers have truly been answered and have blessed Molly! She is awesome! God Bless All Of You!

Lisa

[We have daughters in the same grade and school... this hit her as it would any mom with a child similar in age... her admonishments were greatly appreciated]

To: Cathy
From: David T
Sent: Thursday, July 20

    AMEN

[Note: I look forward to the day that I can say this back to him... he is Rebekah's dad.]

To: Cathy
From: Candy
Sent: Thursday, July 20

WOW! Praise God. I'm calling you now.

Love,
Candy

[This is my friend in San Antonio... she is not much for the Internet but I can't tell you how many times she talked me through anxious thoughts on the phone. She knew just when to call... guess she was listening as God whispered.]

To: Cathy
From: Carolyn F
Sent: Thursday, July 20

I have been thinking of you all day long. What a joyous email read for me and for all. Cathy, words can never express the feelings and thoughts of those you have touched... and you and Molly have touched so many! The tears of joy are flooding the Internet this day... What a sight that must have been with the precious Jodeit family 'looking on' as Molly rang the bell. Tell Molly that the bell must have been heard by everyone who has been touched by her story. I am so happy and so elated for all of you. What an incredible journey you have taken us through. Now, if you and Kitty would just keep up those daily devotionals... God must be so proud of all you... His angels on earth. I am certain that He was also watching Molly ring that bell. Love and hugs, and more hugs to all.

To: Cathy
From: Mel
Sent: Thursday, July 20

Your excellent message brought more tears to my eyes. Isn't it amazing that at the beginning of this year, Molly's health was not at the top of our wish list, but after her diagnosis of cancer, it quickly took the top spot. It just goes to show that we generally take for granted the most valuable gifts that God has bestowed upon us. I thank God for the health and well being of our entire family and ask that it is His will that this will continue through eternity...

To: Cathy
From: Jo Ann
Sent: Thursday, July 20

Dearest Cathy,

YEA! Molly has rung the bell and it is over! I prayed for her all day today! Thank you so much for sharing today with all of us and for sharing Molly's whole journey with us. When I read your e-mail I could close my eyes and see the huge SMILES that were on each of your faces as you celebrated with her! What PRAISE TO THE LORD! And what a BLESSING and a PRIVILEGE to have been one of her many prayer warriors. I will continue to lift her up in prayer as well as you and Mel and your whole family.

Cathy, the Lord really used YOU in a mighty way through all of this. You are and have always been one of His "SPECIAL AMBASSADORS." He has used you in so many different ways to bring others to Him, this was just one of HIS BIG WAYS TO USE YOU and you said "yes" and took the challenge. The Lord is in the business of "changing hearts" and we are but His instruments. You were indeed His instrument spreading His Word to everyone, from your family to all of us to everyone at the hospital. We have all been so RICHLY BLESSED and I know that you and everyone in your whole family have, too. Thank you for your "boldness in the Lord" and for not only sharing your faith in Him, but your feelings and emotions throughout this journey. We "can do all things through Him who strengthen us" if we let Him be our guide and that you all did. I'm sure that the Lord is smiling up in His Heavenly realms and saying "Well done, good and faithful servant." I love you...

jo ann

[I have not changed one tiny part of this email so that you could see the expression of love and faithfulness that is so noted here.]

To: Cathy
From: Gene and Shelley
Sent: Thursday, July 20

Thank you for this wonderful uplifting message of faith and trust. The Lord is good and faithful and Shelley & I, our whole family, rejoice with you. We love you guys. Give Molly a hug from some of her biggest fans, the J's...

[Note: We used to have a little group of four couples that would go to dinner together once a month. The J's and The Jodeit's are the only ones left in town... so when we would go to dinner, Molly got stuck coming with us. The J's have a vested interest in Molly for she was part of our dinner group for many years.... then she started driving and bowed out... imagine that... better things to do.]

To: Cathy
From: Kay S
Sent: Friday July 21

I know this "Thanksgiving feast" held more thanks than you knew imaginable and I am so proud of the Jodeit family—you have truly let God turn lemons into lemonade in front of more people than I can begin to count. Way to go Molly.

From,
Kay

To: Cathy
From: Jill
Sent: Sunday, July 23

Cathy, just another thought about prayer. In John 14:13-14,

John 15:16b, John 16:23b-24 and numerous other references, Jesus is categorically insisting that we pray and that we pray in His name, and He promises us that He will grant our requests. The key here is asking in Jesus' name, because when we truly pray in His name, we are praying the prayer that Jesus would pray.

How do we know how Jesus would pray? By knowing Him so intimately through His Word. I am so thankful for His powerful answers to our prayers for Molly. He has been glorified and has changed all of our lives forever. He has really ministered to me through you, Cathy. Press on, my friend. I am one of your many "balcony people" applauding both Him and you.

In His arms of love,
Jill

To: Cathy
From: Jan C
Sent: Sunday, July 23

BELLS ARE RINGING IN MY HEART FOR YOU. I DON'T HAVE THE WORDS TO TELL YOU HOW I AM FEELING, BUT TEARS ARE STREAMING! LOVE YOU!

Jan

[I know this to be true... for she is my crying angel]

To: Cathy
From: Kitty
Sent: Sunday, July 23

I had tears of joy reading this. Wish I could have been there.

Love,
Kitty

[What a true blessing and lightening rod she has been... God's smile is upon her... good job, faithful servant!]

To: Cathy
From: Cathy and Bill
Sent: Monday, July 24

Cathy and I can't tell you how happy we were to hear about the bell ringing—with all that it means—for Molly's courage and her family's support and faith. Molly is half-way through high school but for me she will always be my little fishing partner at Camp Mystic. Please give her our very best wishes. We look forward to seeing you all the in the months ahead. You are wonderful people and very special friends.

Love,
Cathy and Bill

[We became friends with Cathy and Bill through our daughters who were in high school together. These have been some of Molly's greatest fans since she was a little girl. Molly and Bill became fast friends when Jennifer and their only daughter Elizabeth went to camp together. When our families stayed in the same motel on the river for camp pick ups, Bill would take Molly fishing with him... she loved it! And loved him! Molly was the little one everyone loved to love when we went for camp pick up!]

To: Cathy
From: Lindy
Sent: Monday, July 24

Woke up thinking about you and Molly and your family this morning. I hope you can rest and enjoy just being home. I do remember feeling that being home is such a luxury and that feeling has never left me. I LOVE being home—I have almost become a recluse, but a very happy one.

I have sent you something that you should receive in the mail. I do NOT want a thank you note. Just email me to let me know that you got it. You need to spend your time being with your girl and being with God and not writing silly thank you notes. Your thank you note is letting us all share your journey. It has been so special and I feel so blessed for getting to be a part of it, even at a distance. You and Molly have touched so many lives. Many thanks.

Love you dear Cathy,
Lindy

[A SPECIAL NOTE HERE regarding the above e-mail: When we got home from ringing the bell at Methodist…the bell rang at my house and this package was delivered via the post office… The irony: The gift Lindy had sent was a large charger sized plate she had hand painted and had written the following inscription on: "PRAISE GOD WHEREVER YOU ARE OR WHATEVER SITUATION HE HAS ALLOWED YOU TO BE IN…HIS GLORY WILL SHINE THROUGH"…all I could do was cry, hold the plate to my chest and say "THANK YOU, LORD"…for only God could nudge the perfect friend, to bestow the perfect gift at the perfect time. It was the exclamation point of a God driven journey! What a blessing! It was finished!…And GOD'S GLORY WAS SHINING!

Thank you Lindy for my plate and for sending God's message in such a beautiful package.]

To: Molly's Prayer Warriors
From: Cathy
Sent: Wednesday, July 26
Subject: Molly PICC line

May I just ask one more specific prayer for Molly—the last procedure we have to do is to get this PICC line taken out. Today we were at the hospital from 9—4 and there were complications and we will go back tomorrow morning at 9:00 to try to complete the process. Her muscles have grabbed hold and will not release the line. Please pray that after 24 hours her body will regroup and it will come out with ease with any further adieu. Thank you so much—every prayer that we have specifically requested has been honored and I trust that God is handling this His way as well!

Cathy

Praise God wherever you are and whatever situation He has allowed you to be in...His glory will shine through!

To: Molly's Prayer Warriors
From: Cathy
Sent: Thursday, July 27
Subject: Trouble with Molly's PICC Line

I have had this Southwest Airlines line in my mind now for days... there is a BELL... then the comments—you are now free to move around the country... same basic line that you get when you're flying and the "fasten your seat belt" light has been turned off, you are now free to move about the cabin. We're rung the BELL. Now we want the freedom! Well, here we are at the end of our trail and with no hitches, which is so unbelievable in itself. Still yesterday, Dr. McClain said this is the FIRST Hodgkin's patient who has not had to be hospitalized during treatment. God's hand was shown. Now all we have left to do is to remove the PICC line. This was supposed to be the easiest part. So, this morning in my quiet time I knew there was a lesson here.

> James 1:25 But the man who looks intently into the perfect law that gives freedom, and continues to do this, not forgetting what he has heard, but doing it—he will be blessed in what he does

FREEDOM: What am I holding so tight to that I have not chosen to release to God or what is holding me so tight that God has no room to move.

Oswald Chambers today said, "God's training is for now, not

later, His purpose is for this very minute, not for sometime in the future. We have nothing to do with what will follow our obedience, and we are wrong to concern ourselves with it.
What people call preparation, God sees as the goal itself.

God's purpose is to enable me to see that He can walk in the storms of my life RIGHT NOW. If we have a further goal in mind, we are not paying enough attention to the present time. However, if we realize moment by moment obedience is the goal, then each moment as it comes is precious.

> What am I holding on to?
> What is holding on to me?
> Who is holding on to me?

In this world that we live in Freedom is dictated by decision making; and who is making the decisions. We adhere to those decisions by our freedom of choice. Obedience reflects submissiveness to somebody else. I so often want to be the one making the decisions, controlling the situation, etc. but I am learning to start thinking differently. Believe me, with my strong WILL this is pretty hard to reevaluate and renegotiate but the way God is helping me to understand this is:

> GOD SEES EVERYTHING—I don't
> GOD KNOWS EVERYTHING—I don't
> GOD IS EVERYWHERE—I am not

So the bottom line here is:

Who is muscling you?
What has hold of you that you are not willing to give it up to God's control? To me, it is my anxiety, my feelings, my family, health, finances. You name it: I am trying to control it! I know that God means for us to enjoy HIM and the Life that He has given us, no matter what our walk. But if I continue to try to muscle GOD and not let God muscle me, I will continue to battle with the Freedom and Joy that God has offered me in my life.

Just like the muscles in Molly's arm, I have to let go to be able to move freely!

Psalm 119:45 I will walk about in FREEDOM, for I have sought out your precepts.

It is God's GLORY that is at stake here. NOT mine—Mine doesn't matter.

Cathy

Praise God wherever you are and whatever situation He has allowed you to be in... His glory will shine through!

To: Molly's Prayer Warriors
From: Cathy
Sent: Thursday, July 27
Subject: Finally FREE FROM PICC Line

SHE IS FREE! Free to wear sleeveless tops, free from daily PICC flushes, free to take a shower, and free from bandages. We went in this morning about 9:00 and about 30 minutes later, it was out! The muscles had relaxed and so had she. When the nurse came in for the procedure, there was no hesitation; the line came out without pause. Again specific prayers were answered! Thank you Dear Friends. She is just relieved... And free... really free!

Cathy

Praise God wherever you are and whatever situation He has allowed you to be in... His glory will shine through!

To: Molly's Prayer Warriors
From: Cathy
Sent: Saturday, July 29
Subject: Bentley Boundaries

During Molly's tackle with cancer, many of you remember that Mel bought her a puppy. Bentley (a name she had picked out since 6th grade... hoping that one day she would have a dog that she could name). Bentley is a yellow lab and sweet temperament, 50 lbs at age 6 months, looks you in the eyes and just loves to be around people.

I have learned a bunch of God's lessons by watching Bentley and the different stages she has wondered through. Last night was one of them. We were having some friends over for dinner. I cleaned the house (piles of paper and magazines that have built up for four months) and Mel came home and said, "I will make you a deal (I have been bugging him for a couple of weeks for Bentley to be able to sleep out of her crate). If you will help me carry the crate to the garage we'll give Bentley a chance to sleep in freedom"... but only one night at a time! THIS WAS A TEST. Of course I complied... The question is "Can we trust her?"

Don't you think that is sometimes the question God is asking us? Can I trust you with this test? Then on faith he sets us up. Gives us a hard lesson and stands back and watches. Bentley knows her spot—we exchanged the crate for a blanket with no boundaries... but she knows that that is her spot. I gave her a chew toy and 3 different times she followed me to my bedroom and 3 times I gently escorted her back to her spot and loved her. The last time she stayed. You know your spot—You are a child of God, You know your boundaries. God very gently works with us to keep us on course one time after another and at some point we finally begin to get it. We STAY in HIS WORD, We STAY UNDER HIS UMBRELLA, and We STAY IN the SPOT he has selected for us to be in.

Can God trust you—are you confident of the spot that you are in with GOD—or do you need a few more nights in the crate? The thing about a crate is it is a secure spot—no one can get in and you sure can't get out. Maybe it' time for you to show God you are trustworthy. The next time you have a storm just assail on your life, TRUST GOD and let Him TRUST YOU. Think about what you know to be true, and WHO you know to be true.

The answer is YES, GOD CAN TRUST YOU... AS LONG AS YOU ARE TRUSTING GOD... it all comes back to God and HIS GLORY!

Bentley was perfect all night—she passed her test—and when morning light came Mel went to see where she had landed (for he still couldn't believe she was even inside she was so quiet). She was in our old dog's bed (Khaki, she starts out in the den and then moves to the living room). In the very room we left her in...calm, confident and very pleased. She didn't know it was a test but she behaved as she had been trained...Am I behaving as I have been trained?

> Psalm 92:1 I will say of the LORD, "He is my refuge and my fortress, my God, in whom I trust."

> This is a trustworthy saying. And I want you to stress these things, so that those who have trusted in God may be careful to devote themselves to doing what is good. These things are excellent and profitable for everyone.

> John 14:1 [Jesus Comforts His Disciples] "Do not let your hearts be troubled. Trust in God; trust also in me.

> OSWALD CHAMBERS SAID July 24th "The only thing that exceeds right doing is right being"

We have just completed the test God gave our family. It was a hard one! No matter how prepared we were it still wasn't enough to "ace" it. We passed no doubt...but only with help, and a bunch of it. We have been blessed in a mighty way by a mighty God.

This was a journey that has taught us many life lessons; those of grace, perspective, love, steadfastness, trust, inadequacies, and FAITH...most of all FAITH in our awesome God. He is who He says He is!!!!! And does what He says He will do! His ways are perfect for us thought we may not see the significance at the time.

Cathy

Praise God wherever you are and whatever situation He has allowed you to be in...His glory will shine through!

Afterword

To: Cathy
From: Wanda
Sent: Thursday, July 27

Woo-hoo! I think we all need to go out and celebrate. I feel like I've been through all this myself. I know we all have felt so personally a part of this journey and have felt the touch of God in our lives through it all. Those private people (and we all know someone who is) who say, "I don't want anyone to know about my struggles," I say, "Look at Molly Jodeit." I'm so glad, Cathy, you didn't deny Molly or your family the joy of being surrounded and lifted up by those who know and love you and trust God with her precious life. That should carry all of you for the rest of your lives. I'm sure God is soooo tired of hearing, "Molly, Molly, Molly." Can we just get on with someone else's life now? :>) There I go with my weird sense of humor. We're so excited for her.

Love,
Wanda

[This was one of my favorite e-mails... to this day I still have the picture that Wanda painted about God hearing the prayers for "MOLLY MOLLY MOLLY" and it warms my heart. For he certainly did hear her name from the thoughts and prayers and lips of so many of you... and he honored your plea for her to be cleared of cancer.]

To: Cathy
From: Kitty
Sent: Thursday, July 27

Praise God from whom all blessings flow! Time to celebrate. When do you leave on your trip?

Kitty

To: Cathy
From: Kay S
Sent: Thursday, July 27

Words cannot tell you how happy I am for that sweet angel as well as all of you. Life is NEVER in our control and this detour just brings it more to the forefront.

God bless you, my sweet friend,
Kay

To: Cathy
From: Ruth Ann
Sent: Thursday, July 27

Praise God!!

Ruth Ann

To: Cathy
From: Kay L
Sent: Thursday July 27

We went to a dinner theater here in Jackson and just loved it. It was

"The Unsinkable Molly Brown." The Molly in the play looked just like you, in coloring, movements. She was darling and very talented. I kept thinking of Molly when she would say, "I'm not down!" She never let anything get her down. I thought of you when she helped the people survive the Titanic and wouldn't let them give up. Her spirit of "can do" reminded me of you and Molly. At the end she missed her "first love" and went back to him. How often do we try to handle everything on our own and finally go back to "our first love?" You never did that from the get go. You always went to HIM and asked others to also. Tell Molly, I will always think of her as "the unsinkable Molly Brown".

[This was also one of my favorites, not that I did not appreciate all of them, I did, we all did…but the "Unsinkable Molly Brown"… our Molly was!]

To: Cathy
From: Kitty
Sent: Wednesday, August 2

Treatment is over. The Jodeit's are celebrating in LA (Molly's choice). Please join me in claiming this verse for Molly: "This trouble will not come a second time on Molly." Nahum 1:9

What a privilege it has been to share this journey. May God abundantly bless Molly, Cathy, Mel, and the entire Jodeit family.

Love,
Kitty

Treatments for this journey began on March 27, 2006 and ended exactly four months later on July 27, 2006. We had no delays, no hospitalizations, only one transfusion between chemo and radiation for security sake (using my blood). We also had an unexpected 9 day early finishing time because Dr. Paulino combined 2 four day field treatments. He also allowed her to waive a regrouping week between radiation fields because her counts were steady.

Yes, God led this expedition... and He conquered our fear with FAITH! We are eternally grateful for His Healing Hand upon Molly and our whole family.

Let me say that these e-mail were only a part of this journey and the support that was given. There are no words to express the appreciation of our whole family for the many gifts and dinners and surprises and phone calls and prayers that were extended to each of us. We were overwhelmed by the love of family, friends, neighbors and acquaintances and will be forever grateful for God's army that you each were a part of. We thank you all from the top of our heads to the tips of our toes.... and deep within the depths of our hearts.

For those of you who have ended up with this little book in your hands... it is by no means an accident. Perhaps you needed encouragement during a hard time, maybe you have never seen or read a real life example of how God works.... or maybe, God just wanted to show you a little glimpse of how you too have the means to invite HIM to be a living part of your life.

There are no magic words or magic ways... God has made it simple... just ask and believe that God is God and it is through the life and death of his son Jesus Christ that he hears our prayers. God willingly and joyfully accepts us as his children.

A storm with God by your side is only a storm,
A storm without God takes a different form.
For with God you are addressing it inside to out,
And without God you are addressing it outside to in! CJodeit

Thank you God.... just Thank you!

As an update on Molly as of June 2007: She is free! The Stanford V protocol that was used for Molly's treatment at Texas Children's Hospital is now being used on other Hodgkin's patients at Texas Children's... and has been successful as well! She blazed a trail for Hodgkin's patients in Houston.

God had a plan for this book well before it was written; for when we were exchanging these frequent e-mails, never did it occur to me that it would ever be published, or that anyone else would want to read this journal of our journey. Many people asked me to continue with the devotionals even though this story was complete.

I accepted the challenge and have continued to write devotionals each weekday and I send them to many of the folks that have followed this journey. A book entitled "Simply God... Encouragement for the Soul" is in current production and is a collection of some of these selected writings.

One thing I have learned about God; he is full of surprises, and when he wants something done... he will do it! I have been blessed that God has inspired my thoughts and pray that he will continue to give me the inclination and motivation to pursue HIS purposes. May His Glory always shine ... through me... and also through you... and the circumstances that he orchestrates.

Rebekah

I know after reading this many will ask about the status of our precious friend Rebekah. She and her family are mentioned several times in this book. The following is a brief synopsis of her cancer journey.

The cancer that she has is called Rabdomyosarcoma. What a huge word and what an obstinate disease. Rebekah began this cancer journey in May 2004. She began with surgery and at that time had several nodules on her neck removed. Following the surgery, the first phase of treatments began and lasted through ten months. They included chemo and were followed by radiation. On the day of her last treatment, she found a spot in her nose. Surgery again was deemed necessary to remove the small tumor. So just a couple of days after her first phase... it all started again. Same routine, but different drugs. She had to again go through nine more months of chemo followed by radiation. The journey was intense and long but finally it had been defeated... or so they thought.

Their freedom lasted only four months. This time that beast of a disease came back in her cheek. Surgery again. Chemo again... June 2006 through October. The chemo wasn't working. Not only was it not working on the existing cancer but new spots were growing. On each occasion a new drug was tried. The drugs which had normally worked on this type of cancer laid down in defeat. November and December 2006 Rebekah was pulled off of everything.

The Clinical Trail Phase One that would have given her an opportunity to try experimental drugs was full. As this is being written in February of 2007, her doctors, Dr. Winston Huh and Dr. Beverly Raney are trying to come up with a combination of drugs that will at least put a HOLD on the cancer until a new drug of promise is found.

This has been a roller coaster of emotions, decisions, celebrations and disappointments for Rebekah and her mom and dad. I only can speak from the standpoint of a mom, and you moms who are reading this will understand. When one of your children is hurting, it absolutely hits you in your gut. You want to shelter them, take it from them, or find a way to minimize the discomfort…and when there is nothing you can do to "make it better"…it is a heart wrenching frustration that no one can soothe but GOD HIMSELF.

Please join us, the Jodeit family and so many others who are lifting this child and her parents up in prayer. I ask that you specifically pray that a new drug will soon come available that will destroy this monster cancer that lurks within Rebekah. Ask God to prepare her body so that when the drug is administered, the effects will be immediate.

Rebekah is now 20 years old. She is a beautiful, confident and a precious child of the Lord. He has used her in his mighty way to proclaim his presence and to tell his story. Through her, others have seen the gentle loving God that she so believes in and has put her faith in. This recurrent cancer has not been a thief of the love and joy that she shares for Lord or for the ones she loves.

Her parents have been valiant warriors as well. They have stood right beside her throughout every moment of this battle. She has been blessed greatly by their presence and their encouragement and their constant desire to make life as best as it could be. The family has also been blessed with wonderful support of friends from all walks of life as well. Their prayer net is as great as the net the fishermen cast out upon the Lord's command…and the prayers that are being lifted up are spilling forth unto our God in Heaven. God has got his hand upon this family in spite of what the world sees on the outside. His plans are perfect and his ways are not our ways. But still I pray, "Please Lord, let this be the year she is healed."

However, if you were to ask Rebekah what she wants you to pray for. It would not be, that she will be healed in a week, a month, or a year; for this is what people prayed for at the beginning of her cancer journey and still three years later she continues to be burdened with this illness. She is a realist, and would want you to pray that God's will be done in her life. She knows that God does not make mistakes and his timing is perfect for His plan for her life.

Before I signed off to the accuracy of this summary, I asked Rebekah to review it... Well, she has read it and she sat by my side as I wrote that last paragraph. Those were HER thoughts. May God keep his hand upon her and fill her with his peace as she continues to fight this stubborn disease. May her courage be steadfast, and may her tenacious spirit be a reflection of her faith in our mighty God.

Thank you

Thank you to you dear readers who have picked this book up. My hope is that the Lord has used some of this to encourage you to walk with him a little closer, or trust him a little more or to encourage you if you just feel like the world around you is crashing down.

We serve a mighty and wonderful God... and I thank God for you... yeah, you... just the way they are!

My prayer for you is this: May your heart be opened so that you may know Jesus and may his love penetrate to your very soul. For the Love of God, who sent His son Jesus to this world to die on our behalf so that we would have everlasting life, is where His Love truly was magnified. This is the love I am asking him to cover you heart and soul with THIS MIGHTY LOVE which knows no bounds.

Amen
Blessings to you my new friends...
For now you too have shared in our story! Thank you!

Things I've Learned as I have journeyed through Molly's cancer...

1) Talk out loud to God immediately–no quiet whispers–ASK HIM FOR HELP NOW
2) Don't panic–there are wonderful Dr.'s–and we live in a city of medical can dos
3) Buy a notebook–one that fits in a purse and a pen that can connect on to it
4) Write down everything–names of nurses, names of Doctors, meds, phone #'s, diagnoses, speculations, fears, prayers, valet #, best friends phone # (because you will find that you will even forget that)
5) Adopt the view of the story of "The Little Train that Could"... think you can and if you can't God will
6) Watch carefully everything the nurses do–just learn—ask questions
7) Have gum–some of the medicines taste awful and the gum curbs it
8) You can have an IV left in over night for a treatment the following day–but you have to fight for it
9) Find out what the main fears of the patient are–Molly's were needles and staying over night in the hospital–She chose a PICC line which eliminated most of the needles and Stanford V (one of the advantages of this protocol was that it eliminated the need for most hospital stays, and the treatment was more condensed thus shorter weeks)–these might not be the case for everyone but for us they worked
10) There is a cover for the PICC line–it costs about $35.00 and you order it over the Internet. The name of the company is Desert Medical Essentials–1–888–215–9545 Molly is a slim, 16 year old and we ordered a size medium, which was perfect.
11) Always take to the infusion:
snacks–sweets usually don't work–small sandwiches do
$1.00 bills for drink machine
Soft blanket–it is cold in the infusion room
12) Try to find someone who has walked this road first–call them We

talked to our friends and this was the information they shared with us:

a) You will get through this

b) God is Big

c) It hurts your heart to watch a child suffer.... beware and ask God for a shield so that you will be fortified to do your best with least emotion

d) Talk to school as soon as possible–she even told me who to talk to because our girls were at the same school

e) Hang out in the Psalms–God will use his word to give you comfort and strength

g) A Bend in the Road is a book by David Jeremiah–helps you see others who identify with your struggles

h) Move a twin bed in your room–we didn't do this but for some reason when she told me this it satisfied my protective, guardianship role knowing that I wouldn't be a sissy if I did—nor would Molly... this is scary and you want to hover under those wings of those who you feel like would protect you–my wings were God's, Molly's were ours!

i) Just take only one day at a time... don't borrow trouble... be prepared, but don't borrow trouble

13) Distractions are good–when chemo is over for the day and if Molly still had energy we did something... anything... that was different. Do whatever it takes to change the focus. Molly and I and Mel usually had lunch and then Molly and I went window shopping or to some retro stores (she loves vintage things). Then her body would wind down and we would go home and she would sleep the rest of the day. As far as a long term distraction–Mel bought her a puppy! This was a wonderful distraction for me too.

14) Take the nausea drugs BEFORE the nausea hits–especially the FIRST 2 weeks, every Monday, Tuesday, Wednesday and Thursday–then you might only need it for a couple of days.

15) Hot baths aren't so good–warm baths are.

16) Chemo seems to have the same results as morning sickness–so go with whatever the craving is just to keep something in her stomach

17) Honor her not wanting to see people–let her do that on her

own timing- don't push any social stuff- remember this is her battle and so many things are OUT OF HER HANDS... let her control the things she is able to.

18) Don't forget to encourage–it is just the little words–you did great today, you look so pretty, I don't know how you are so brave, I'm proud of you, I don't think I would have been able to handle this with as much poise as you have, you have been a great sport, you have great courage, and you are so appreciative... thank you!... or just plain great job! Remind her of what she has already accomplished... you are getting closer toward your goal

19) Siblings are going through this too–keep up with their lives and honor their concerns this is hard because so much of your energies are keeping up with the patient but remember the other siblings need a little encouragement too... I wasn't so good at this.

20) Home care–if you can do it yourself–Do–I had to flush Molly's lines each night with Saline and then Heparin–and have to change her dressing once a week.

When you do it yourself you are on your own schedule–and as far as changing the dressing–she can take as long as she wants to remove the old one–that sometimes hurts and I have all the time in the world if I can take some stress out of this deal. Also, it was nice to NOT have "Someone else" in the picture. You want to "take away" instead of "add to" this deal if you can.

21) The first 2 weeks are the hardest because there is so much anxiety about the unknown; not to mention that there are so many different meds to be taken at home. Jennifer, my daughter made me a spreadsheet of what I needed to do for each day. I needed it the first couple of weeks because I am awful at keeping new schedules and new routines. It was a huge help!

And this is a whole new routine–you'll get the hang of it–it just takes time. Don't panic if your make mistakes... believe me, it happens! I either forgot to give her a dose or gave her two on consecutive days instead of alternating, etc. After confessing to the Dr. he said with the drugs we are taking at home the routine that is structured is best but an occasional accidental diversion won't hurt. Good thing!

22) If you need to cry–just cry–don't hold it in–this journey is hard– and besides I came to the conclusion that the word cry is used so

many times in the bible God expects that of me–but cry to God–you know in Psalm 56 God talks of keeping record of all of your tears… that gave me great freedom.

23) Find someone who will e-mail a list of concerned friends an update; it saves phone calls, lots of visits and keeps family & friends who are praying and concerned up to date

24) Make a medicine chart the first 2 or 3 weeks—what meds what days and keep a record of times meds were given

25) Finally, remember we serve a mighty and faithful God–Trust Him–when doubts start to creep in—PUSH them out with God's promises–only one thought can have access to your mind at a time LET IT BE POSITIVE—God's love is encompassing—embrace it!

26) I bought a Life Application bible and had Molly's name engraved on it—I underlined each verse that people would send me who were praying for her as well as verses I would fine. She hasn't opened it yet but one day I think it will be a treasure

27) Take one day at a time—just one day… before you know it you will be down the road looking back counting your blessings.

28) Attitudes are contagious—BE POSITIVE—Molly is reading me and taking cue cards from what I think and how I respon—Yikes!

29) Say thank you—to the Doctors, to the staff, to your husband, to your kids, to your friends—we're all pulling this wagon together!

30) Always have HOPE—no matter what! It helped me to keep HOPE in my heart; C.A.N.C.E.R.—Christ Always Negotiates Circumstances for Eternal Riches for He will take care of this!

Thank you Lord for placing your healing hand on our Molly and for the blessing of being able to share her story and show your Glory throughout our journey.

Amen.

Contact Cathy Jodeit at cathyjodeit.com